life balance

life balance

the essential keys to a lifetime of well-being

HEATHER MILLS McCARTNEY AND BEN NOAKES

MICHAEL JOSEPH
an imprint of
PENGUIN BOOKS

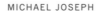
MICHAEL JOSEPH

Published by the Penguin Group
Penguin Books Ltd, 80 Strand, London WC2R 0RL, England
Penguin Group (USA) Inc., 375 Hudson Street, New York, New York 10014, USA
Penguin Group (Canada), 90 Eglinton Avenue East, Suite 700, Toronto, Ontario, Canada M4P 2Y3
(a division of Pearson Penguin Canada Inc.)
Penguin Ireland, 25 St Stephen's Green, Dublin 2, Ireland (a division of Penguin Books Ltd)
Penguin Group (Australia), 250 Camberwell Road,
Camberwell, Victoria 3124, Australia (a division of Pearson Australia Group Pty Ltd)
Penguin Books India Pvt Ltd, 11 Community Centre,
Panchsheel Park, New Delhi – 110 017, India
Penguin Group (NZ), cnr Airborne and Rosedale Roads, Albany,
Auckland 1310, New Zealand (a division of Pearson New Zealand Ltd)
Penguin Books (South Africa) (Pty) Ltd, 24 Sturdee Avenue,
Rosebank, Johannesburg 2196, South Africa

Penguin Books Ltd, Registered Offices: 80 Strand, London WC2R 0RL, England

www.penguin.com

First published 2006
1

Grateful acknowledgement is made for permission to quote on page 83
the concept of K. Bradford Brown Ph.D., and to reproduce 'Time Tested Beauty Tips' from
In One Era And Out The Other by Samuel Levenson, reprinted by permission of SII/Sterling
Lord Literistic, Inc., copyright 1973 by Samuel Levenson

*The information in this book is intended for informational purposes only, and will be
relevant to the majority of people but may not be applicable in each individual case. The book
is sold with the understanding that neither the publisher nor the authors are engaged in
rendering financial, medical or other professional services in publishing this book. Neither the
publishers nor the authors can accept responsibility for any personal injury or other damage
or loss arising from the use or misuse of the information and advice in this book, or
arising out of a failure by a reader to take medical or other professional advice.*

Set in 10.5/16 pt MT News Gothic
Typeset by Rowland Phototypesetting Ltd, Bury St Edmunds, Suffolk
Printed in Great Britain by Clays Ltd, St Ives plc

A CIP catalogue record for this book is available from the British Library

ISBN-13: 978–0–718–14667–2
ISBN-10: 0–718–14667–0

Contents

LIFE BALANCE

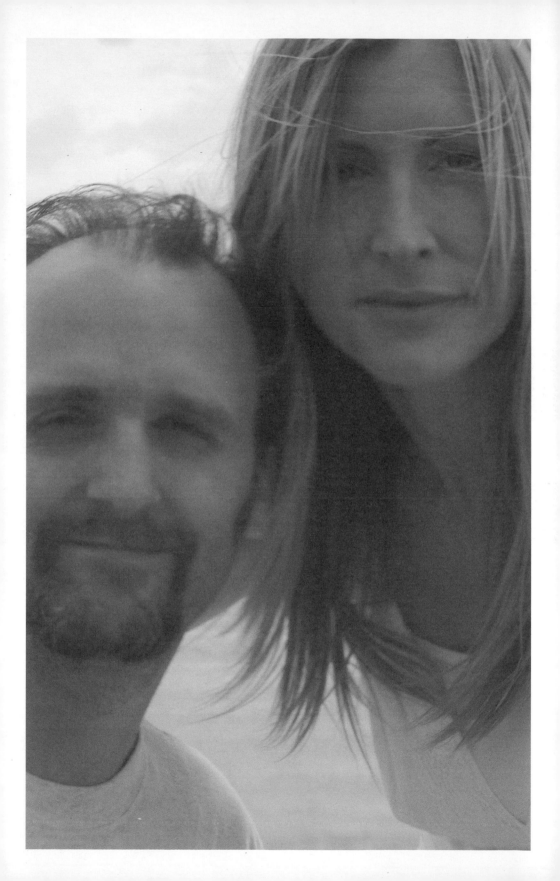

Life Balance

An Introduction

Heather: *We all need to balance the practical elements of a busy life – family, friends, career – but finding and maintaining equilibrium in life is about more than that. It is also about balancing our physical, emotional and spiritual lives. Over the years I have had periods of affluence and times of near penury, times of good health and times of injury and illness. I have learnt that peace of mind has very little to do with luxury or leisure.*

Ben: *Heather and I have been friends for over ten years. When we first met I was setting up an independent TV production company in London, and the BBC asked us to make a series of films featuring Heather interviewing celebrities on how they chill out. At that time in my life I guess I was a fairly ambitious and superficial person. I measured success largely in terms of material possessions and career prestige – the house, the car, that sort of thing. One of the things that immediately struck me about Heather was her lack of interest in these things yet, seven or eight years later when my business collapsed, taking with it the things I had most valued, Heather was the best friend I could have wished for. She even offered to pay my bills until I was back on my feet again. I have learnt through the intervening* *years that happiness is an elusive concept if you try to find it outside of yourself. It's an inside job, and at the end of the day this comes down to finding some measure of harmony in your life.*

Heather: *Life has an uncanny knack of throwing us all off-balance from time to time – from the smallest thing that seems like nothing to someone else, to major life crises that threaten everything we thought we knew about ourselves. I literally lost my balance when I lost my leg; Ben lost his when he lost his business. What I am sure of is that when we achieve and maintain equilibrium in our everyday lives, the punches that life throws no longer feel as though they will overthrow our whole life, they are simply other challenges to be met. Our intention in writing this book is to lay out a set of tools which can be used by anyone – the essential keys for life balance – and to provide you with the confidence to take any of these tools and find out more about them.*

Ben: *Take these tools and use them well, together they will provide you with the basic building blocks that you need. Enjoy them through life's highs and come back to them when you lose your way and you feel the balance of your life is disrupted.*

How do you define 'success'? Are you essentially materialistic, interpreting success in terms of material or career achievement? Or is spiritual fulfilment your only goal? Often we have an image of ourselves that suggests we care as much for our emotional or spiritual development as we do about financial security but, when it comes down to it, the facts indicate otherwise.

Life Balance. An Introduction

It's not really surprising that we sometimes feel confused. Contemporary Western society measures success in terms of accomplishing certain tasks rather than how we **feel**. To describe someone as 'successful' almost invariably relates to their actions – to the size of their new house or the status of their job. It is often seen as merely self-indulgent for someone to strive after a sense of well-being and happiness rather than material success. Yet few things matter more than happiness in our lives and the lives of those we love, and few things are as comprehensively ignored by our society as the pursuit of happiness.

Life Balance is an **activity** book in the truest sense of the word. It contains a number of exercises, some of which you will need a pen and paper for. We would suggest that you buy yourself a journal or notebook, one you really like the look of, and use it for all the written exercises and any other thoughts and feelings you have as you work your way through this book. We suggest that you focus your attention on one section at a time and allow yourself sufficient time to absorb the changes in each chapter before moving on to the next.

Be kind to yourself. We have found that taking care of yourself is the greatest gift you can give, not just to yourself but to those around you. This is not a race. As you work through the sections of this book you are laying down roots which can remain in place for a lifetime, allowing you to grow into a happier, more fulfilled and stronger person, and consequently a better mother, brother, friend or lover.

The different sections of this book do not stand alone, each section impacts on the others. When you put in place simple ways to organize your day you may instantly find you have released time to take up exercise. You begin to feel fitter

3

and wish to eat a healthier diet. As a result you have more energy and you go through the chores of the day much more quickly, releasing even more time for yourself. You are able to use this time to consider your emotional and spiritual needs and you begin to feel more confident, more certain of the direction your life is taking. With this certainty comes a greater clarity about what is important, and you are able to prioritize your day more effectively so that you can fulfil more of your emotional needs. And so on, and so on.

Changing your habits is an ongoing process that requires long-term dedication and determination. It's all very well changing your eating patterns, for example, or taking up exercise but once your initial enthusiasm has waned you will find yourself drawing on resources deep within yourself in order to keep on going.

Heather: *We are not here to tell you* **what** *to do* **when**. *Each of us has the power and the strength to change the things we don't like in our lives for the better. The tools in this book will help you but the best part of all is that you do the rest for yourself. This book is just a starting point.*

Ben: *I love the phrase 'attraction rather than promotion' – the idea that you lead by example rather than by persuasion. You can't fix people, in other words. For instance, if Heather had taken me to one side when we first met and suggested I was too materialistic, I would have told her where to go!*

Heather: *A conscious decision is called for in order for us to* **be** *happy. Anyone who wants to achieve any measure of sustained happiness must be prepared to make it a priority in their lives.*

Life Balance. An Introduction

You cannot achieve anything like your full potential for happiness if your self-esteem is low, or if you are in a poor state of physical or emotional health. This is the focus of Life Balance.

The first essential key to a lifetime of well-being:

GET ORGANIZED!

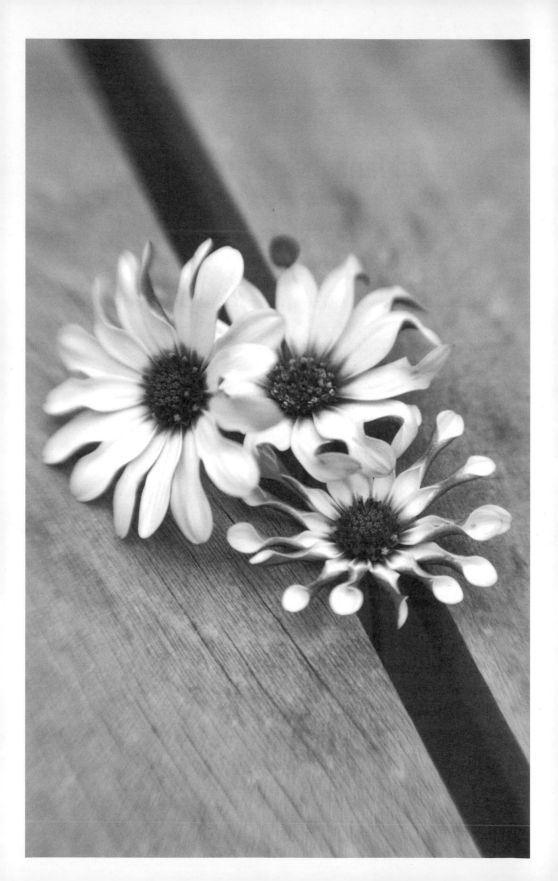

1 | Managing Your Life

Heather: *I really believe that no matter how many aspects there are to your life and how much you have to juggle, it is possible to keep on top of things and maintain balance so long as you manage your life effectively. Life management really comes down to prioritizing your objectives, large and small.*

Ben: *Eight or nine years ago, Heather and I shared an office space in London. Anyone coming in might have been struck by the contrast in our working styles. Whereas Heather was super-efficient, I was always a bit disorganized. I remember once we were filming a television interview about fifty miles outside London, I was co-producing the film and Heather was the interviewer. I'm ashamed to say that I waited until we were driving down the motorway before I checked the map to see where we were going. As a result we arrived ninety minutes late and were greeted by a grumpy film crew and interviewee. I now use some of Heather's time-management skills!*

Heather: *Getting organized and creating a perimeter fence around your space and time is an essential skill for anyone to learn, and it is an ongoing process throughout life. I used to* *agree to all sorts of commitments but my responsibilities soon began to overpower me. When our daughter was born I recognized that if I was going to continue to do the things I enjoy, such as seeing my friends, having time with my husband, going to the gym and also focusing on my work, I would have to learn to balance all these different elements of my life. I now prioritize much more carefully and try to choose what is really important to me. I'm learning to say 'no' to things even though it means disappointing others from time to time.*

It doesn't take much for life to feel overcrowded and out of balance. When was the last time you undertook a proper review of your lifestyle? If your answer is 'Not for a while,' or 'Never,' then read on! The first key to life balance is taking control of the life you have right now.

If you ask a cross-section of people what causes them the greatest stress in their lives most of them will tell you that they simply have too much to do. There's no doubt that some of us actually get off on a little bit of anxiety and without realizing it we can become stress junkies. If you are busy, forever rushing from one task to the next, your body releases the same 'feel-good' chemicals that are released during exercise. If you maintain a busy lifestyle for long enough you might even become chemically dependent on your stress drugs. In this way, many busy people actually welcome their hectic lifestyles, finding it difficult to relax during down time.

It is important that you don't kid yourself that you're getting lots done simply because you are busy. If you have poor time management skills, it might be that you're rushing from one task to the next without achieving very much at all. If this is the case, it's time to get organized!

Activity Log

Your day seems to be chock-a-block full of things to be done. Once the household chores have been completed and the most pressing bills paid, you scarcely have the time (or energy) for anything and end up flopping in front of the telly. You feel you don't have a minute to yourself.

A useful tool in this situation is an activity log, which is a record of how you really spend your time. Carry a small notebook with you wherever you go and write down everything you do. Every time you change your activity, for any reason, make a note of it. Also make a note of times during the day when you feel at your most alert or tired. Your activity log will help you to identify low yield or time-wasting jobs, and it should also alert you to the times when you are at your most productive.

The reality of most people's lives is constant distraction and interruption. Recent studies suggest that some business managers can expect to do six minutes of uninterrupted work at a time. The same applies to many people's domestic lives, particularly if we live with a partner or children. Even if you live alone you may discover through your activity log that you allow yourself to become distracted very easily.

Stick to writing your activity log for a week. At the end of the week take a look at what you spent your time doing.

- How much time did you spend on low yield jobs that did not need to be done?
- Did you allocate appropriate time to the important tasks?
- We all need a break, but how much time did you spend

surfing the net, watching mediocre television shows or chatting around the coffee machine?

- Did you spend more time than you thought clearing up after members of your family, washing their dishes or putting dirty clothes in the laundry basket?
- How much time did you have to yourself and how did you use it?

Lack of planning, poor organization and loose boundaries can make anyone's day a clutter of menial tasks and chores. To get organized we need to set goals and eliminate the things that waste our time.

'To Do' Lists

Heather: *Every morning, except for weekends and holidays, I draw up a job list. Routine is a valuable tool when it comes to managing your time effectively and it is useful to know that at a certain time each day you will be going for a run, for example, or exercising or meditating. Because these take place at fixed times each day, I no longer put them on my 'to do' list. Instead, I use it to prioritize tasks which are not a daily occurrence: phoning a particular client, for example, or replying to an e-mail. Since I became a mum my brain seems to stay in bed some days so I have started to keep a diary as well. I'm also learning the importance of asking for help from others, which many of us don't find easy.*

There are many ways of structuring a 'to do' list and it won't be difficult to find one which suits you. The standard method is to take a new sheet of paper each morning and write down all of your tasks. Break larger jobs down into their component parts and then prioritize your tasks by underscoring or highlighting the most urgent jobs with a highlighter pen. At the foot of the page make a note of any appointments you have so that all your tasks and commitments are on a single sheet of paper. Use your common sense and adapt your tasks to suit your energy levels. Many people feel tired in the middle of the afternoon so don't decide to make all your important phone calls then, do something less demanding instead. Roll up your sleeves and set to it, crossing out the tasks as you complete them.

Some low priority jobs may not need to be addressed for weeks or even months. Write these in an A4 notebook and periodically read through the jobs on this list to see if any should be dealt with now.

If you don't have enough time to complete all the tasks on your daily 'to do' list, so be it. Used properly, your list can be a valuable tool to make your life easier but it is not a weapon to beat yourself up with.

Gradually, windows will begin to appear in an otherwise cluttered day. You will soon be able to make time for yourself where previously even a few moments of peace and inactivity seemed too much to ask.

The Golden Hour

Each of us, if we structure our lives properly, can find a little free time to devote to ourselves. How much time we can carve out of a busy day depends not only on our ability to structure each day effectively but also, of course, on our circumstances. With some careful management, for many of us it should be possible to set aside a whole hour each day – a 'Golden Hour' – entirely for ourselves.

Selfish as it sounds, this daily window will raise your self-esteem and your sense of well-being, and this in turn will filter down to the people closest to you. Who wouldn't benefit from having a happy and zestful wife, husband, son or colleague?

Here's how it works:

As we will be seeing in the course of this book, a daily yoga session can work wonders for your energy, appearance and your self-esteem. The same is true of meditation. Combine these with an exercise routine and you have a perfect foundation for healthy living. These practices complement each other perfectly, leading to a state of equilibrium – balance – catering to the needs of your body, mind and soul.

Making the transition from your life as you experience it now to a healthy, balanced lifestyle isn't easy, of course, but it's your choice. Nobody else can make you feel great. Break it in gradually, perhaps with a few minutes of yoga practice every couple of days and slowly increase this to a daily fifteen-minute session. You can then introduce a meditation session, beginning with five minutes of visualization. Exercise is the big one, not just in terms of the immediate benefits it can bring but also in terms of the amount of effort required to get into it. So the usual rule applies: break it in gently. Don't go off the deep end. Just a few minutes every couple of days is plenty until your body gets used to the new routine.

Making Boundaries

Boundary setting is imperative if you are to be successful in managing your life. It is all very well telling people to put their clothes in the laundry basket but old habits die hard and within a week you might find yourself clearing up after everyone as you have always done. Take control of the situation: 'A new house rule is that everybody clears up after themselves.' Or perhaps you find yourself drifting back into old habits of pottering around not doing much in particular when your activity log has shown that this is by far the most expensive use of your time. Make a mental note of habits like this which need to be avoided and **stick to it**! At work, do you agree to do jobs which are not your concern, taking on other people's responsibilities? Set your boundaries, be firm and learn to say 'no'. You may be surprised how much effort is needed to change the simplest habits but, if you are clear in your intentions and are prepared to make the effort, the benefits will be worthwhile.

This is really a matter of clearly defining boundaries for yourself: 'I will not waste time surfing the net when I should be working,' and for those around you; 'I'll be meditating every day at this time. Please don't interrupt me.' Our own innate laziness means that you will probably be testing your boundaries within a matter of days – 'Maybe just this once . . .' – whereas those around you are likely to see how far they can bend the new rules, whether this is at home or in the office. Be firm. It really is that simple.

If you hit a problem go back to your activity log. See if all the tasks listed are absolutely necessary and whether they can be undertaken in a more time-efficient way. Can technology take the place of manual labour and free up a bit of extra time? Can jobs be delegated? Are you taking on too many responsibilities where you would be better off saying 'no' once in a while? Have you adjusted tasks to your energy levels? Have you broken down large or unwieldy jobs? Are you trying to do too many things at the same time? Are you aiming for perfection, where you might be better off settling for steady progress? Are you keeping enough time in hand each day to handle unexpected complications? These questions are the nuts and bolts of time management; they are there to help you make your daily routine work like a well-oiled machine!

If, when you have whittled essential tasks down to a bare minimum, you find that there's still scarcely a moment free in the day, let alone a golden hour, you might want to consider creating extra productive time by getting up an hour earlier.

Heather: *As a working wife and mother, I have learnt that setting the alarm thirty minutes earlier each morning can make all the difference. It allows me a little bit of personal space before the day begins. I organize everything for breakfast the night before so that I can get it ready without a panic and we can eat together as a family.*

Over the course of a year, getting up an hour earlier effectively creates ten additional weeks. If you decide to get up earlier in the morning you might find it difficult at first but the tiredness will soon pass. If this is impossible for you, don't panic. The great thing about discretionary tasks such as exercise, yoga and meditation is that you can get great results even if you spend just a few minutes on them daily. Remember to factor in a little time just to flop and do nothing, and don't be too hard on yourself if there just aren't enough minutes in the day to squeeze in everything you would like to do.

Ben: *Whereas Heather's a lark, I'm most definitely a night-owl. I hate getting up early and I come alive at about six o'clock most evenings. I tend to start work a little later each morning and finish later in the evening, perhaps at seven-thirty or eight o'clock. There's something cruel about getting up when it's still dark and I try to avoid the experience wherever possible! I have found it works best for me to organize my time and my work around my energy levels.*

Life Goals

A journey of a thousand miles begins with a single step. Once you've organized your time more effectively, the next step in your transition is to answer a simple question: 'What are your priorities?' When we are constantly running to catch up with ourselves we often lose sight of what it is we are working towards. Ask yourself what it is you want out of life. The time management skills outlined in this chapter are not only useful to get you through your day, you can also use them to help you achieve the really big goals in life.

Take a few moments to really consider your goals. Write them down. Do you want a larger house? That sounds reasonable enough, but before committing yourself to this goal, ask yourself what your **motivation** is for wanting it. Could it be that you are looking for the esteem of others in order to feel good about yourself? Once again, this sounds fair enough – after all we all do it – but is there an easier way to achieve a sense of security and well-being? Might you be better off focusing your energies on building up your self-esteem? What would make you feel good **about yourself**? Living a useful and contented life? Not being ashamed of who or what you are? Allowing time for yourself, to nurture yourself and be more aware of your inner needs? Or perhaps taking more care of others? Happiness can take many forms and not all of them come in the shape of houses.

Be precise. Instead of writing, 'I want to feel good,' and leaving it at that, think about how you are going to achieve this – modifying your diet, for example, or letting go of a relationship which is harmful to you. And try to be positive. If you are tempted to write down, 'Stop looking such a ghastly mess all the time,' stop and think. Instead put, 'Make the most of my best features.'

Be realistic, too. There is little point in trying to be an Olympic pentathlete at 52. If you aim too high you will probably be forced to give up, which may lead to the whole edifice crashing down. But by the same token don't aim too low. People tend to do this if they are a little lazy or if they're afraid of failure. Aim to **stretch** your comfort-zone without breaking it altogether.

Take a good look at your list. Are these **your** goals? Do you really want to be a doctor, a lawyer, an accountant? Parents, friends and partners can hoist on to us what they want us to achieve, often without our even being aware of it. Many people get married and try to have children as a matter of course, without stopping to think if it is right for them. Others might fail to pursue careers in the arts or entertainment because family members encourage them to get 'real' jobs. On a smaller scale, could it be that you are held back from making changes in your life – from your eating habits to your hairstyle – because you are concerned that others might disapprove? Perhaps there's a pole-dancer, a punk or a vegetarian lurking a little way beneath the surface, too afraid to come out. By the same token, perhaps you have had enough of living a laid-back lifestyle and have a strong compulsion to don a suit and train in accountancy. Have a bit of fun exploring what changes you would make to your life if nobody were ever to find out. Ask yourself, 'If I could be anybody, do anything, without risk of being caught, what would I be?' You may be surprised by the answers.

Prioritize Your Goals

Once you have completed your list, draw up a fresh one prioritizing your goals. 'Be a better parent' and 'tidy the fridge' may both appear on the same sheet of paper but this doesn't mean that they are of equal significance. Focus on the most important items and don't suffocate yourself with too many objectives. Drop anything from the list which, on reflection, isn't so important. It might simply belong on your long-term 'to do' list.

As we have already seen, the best way to approach any large task is to break it down into smaller, more manageable pieces. With a lifetime's wish list, you might want to draw up a five-year plan, a one-year plan and a one-month plan, thereby creating progressively smaller goals. In this way, even the biggest lifetime task can be broken down into a series of attainable objectives.

You may, for example, dream of dispensing with your job and setting up your own business. The first step towards achieving this could be to undertake a feasibility study. Perhaps your circumstances make this impossible for the next few months so choose a time to do it later in the year and put it on your one-year plan. In the meantime, though, you can get a feel for the competition and this is something you can begin in the next week. In this way you can build up a set of long-, medium- and short-term targets. By rationalizing them effectively (and don't forget to implement your targets) you will find yourself moving towards your goals.

One key advantage of breaking long-term objectives down into short-term goals is that it puts you on the spot as to how you are going to achieve your targets. If a general priority in your life is 'I want to be healthier,' then your short-term strategies can help you decide precisely how you are going to achieve this:

- One-month plan: Improve my diet.
- Three-month plan: Build up daily exercise routine from five minutes to half an hour.

And so on. Periodically review your goal sheet. How are you getting on? Are you achieving your short-term objectives or were they unrealistic? What modifications, if any, should you be making to your long-term plan in response to what you have achieved through your short-term plan?

Most of us are unaware of the extent to which our lives might be improved by even a small amount of restructuring. Now is your opportunity to discover just how cluttered your time and priorities have become. To-do lists, activity logs and prioritizing your goals are simple to implement and their benefits can be both immediate and far-reaching.

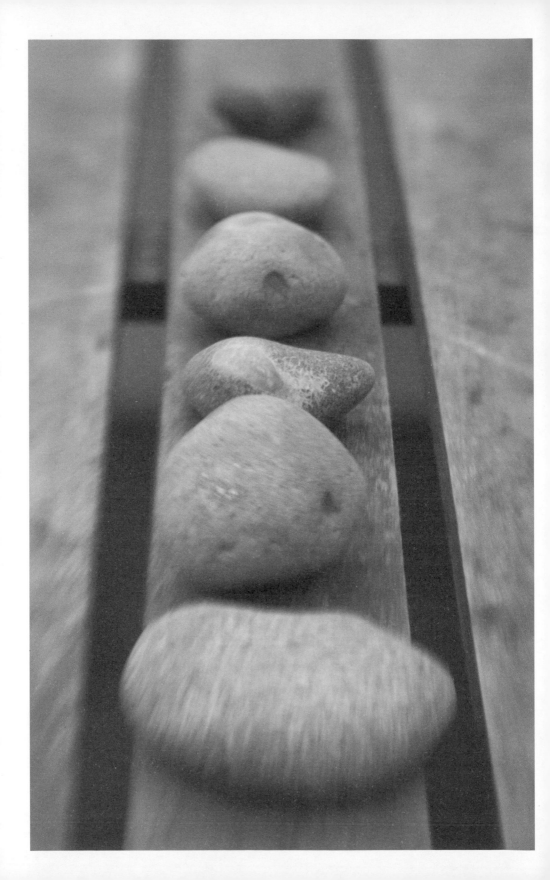

2 | Creating a Positive Environment

Heather: *Almost anywhere can be made into a life enhancing, nurturing space. Natural light, fresh air, a careful choice of colours, flowers – I love the sight and smell of a beautiful bouquet of freshly cut flowers, even the most lacklustre hotel room or office can be transformed with one – do not cost much money but we often underestimate the significant effect these things can have on our mood and happiness. A happy household leads to a positive atmosphere in a building. We've all had a gut instinct about a place – good or bad – that has had nothing to do with the wall hangings or the shade of the carpet. Happy people make a happy home.*

Ben: *I've never been particularly bothered about creating a positive atmosphere with flowers, for example. I suspect that this is a gender thing. Women tend to be better at creating positive, nurturing environments – or am I being sexist? After Heather and Paul were married I noticed a transformation in their home: light pastel fabrics and paintwork, large bunches of flowers on the hall table, and it was wonderful. It really struck me how important it is to create a positive environment. Space, like time, is a precious commodity. For most of us the problem isn't a lack* *of space, it's too much clutter. I used to live in a five-bedroomed Georgian house full of clutter; I now live in a simple but lovely room and I much prefer it, even if I still haven't stretched myself to buying a bunch of flowers. Instead, I got rid of every non-essential thing. Old chairs, teapots and clothing all ended up sitting on the garden wall outside the apartment block and it was great to see it all disappear. Not only did I free up space in my room but I had a tremendous sense of liberation, of letting go of my old life and moving forwards.*

Heather: *This book is partly about identifying those aspects of your life which aren't so good and then dispensing with them. Few endeavours express this purpose more clearly than clearing out the clutter from your home; it is an extremely effective way of creating a sense of new beginnings. In this chapter we will be looking at ways of creating more space by streamlining and prioritizing possessions and making the most of the space you already have. Once you have cleared out your cupboards, attic and boxes, it is then time to create the sort of environment you would like to live in.*

A few centuries ago most people could store everything they owned in a single box or trunk. Nowadays, many of us have so much stuff lurking in the back of cupboards and at the bottom of drawers that we no longer know exactly what we own. One thing is certain: almost all of us would benefit from streamlining our possessions.

Getting Started

Start off by identifying key trouble-spots. Walk around with an A4 pad and a pen. Allowing a separate sheet for each room, make a note of the spaces – a shelf, a cupboard, a particular room – which need your attention.

Next find seven large boxes or bags and a rubbish sack. Mark them as follows:

1. **Put Away** for items that already have a place.
2. **Create a Place** for items you want to keep, but don't yet have a home for.
3. **Action** for letters you need to reply to and suchlike.
4. **Repair** for things that need cleaning, altering or fixing.
5. **Pass On** for items which you can give to charity, sell on eBay or give to a friend.
6. **Recycle**.
7. **Unsure** for items you are undecided about.

Begin on those parts of the house which will give you the greatest reward for the least amount of effort. Throwing out a few newspapers and magazines lying around in the sitting room may take no more than a few minutes but the effects will be immediately obvious. Going through a pile of receipts in the back of a drawer, however, might feel like it takes for ever. Leave the most painstaking tasks until last.

Store away archive material which is not regularly needed. Go through kitchen cupboards and throw away old food tins and rarely used pots and pans. Seek out obsolete medicines from your bathroom cupboard and toys in the attic that are no longer wanted. Take disused keys off your key ring. Empty out your briefcase or handbag and bin scraps of paper and broken pens. As you complete each task tick it off the list.

One of the potential pitfalls in clearing out your clutter is getting waylaid, particularly with interesting paperwork or old photographs. It is easy to lose whole hours in this way if you are not very careful. Put all of these on one side to look at later, perhaps at the end of the day as you relax.

Your home may contain a few items you would be better off without in the long term but you are not yet ready to dispose of. For instance, fluorescent strip-lights can cause headaches and drowsiness and the light they give off is harsh and uninteresting. Rather than immediately going to the trouble and expense of having them removed, pay a visit to a household store like Ikea and invest in some inexpensive table lamps. Over time you can phase out items and appliances which no longer fit into your lifestyle. For now the watchword is progress, not perfection.

You can afford to be quite ruthless when you are clearing out but there are bound to be some difficult calls. It may be that you are nervous of getting rid of a gift you don't like. Taste is a very personal thing and even our nearest and dearest don't always get it right! If you decide to hang on to something you're not wild about, try to find a discreet place for it.

Go through your clothes. If you have two or more of the same thing, keep the newest or best one. If you haven't worn something for a year, get rid of it. If it no longer fits, get rid of it. If it is uncomfortable, get rid of it.

Put items you are not sure about into your 'Unsure' box and store it at the back of a cupboard for a year. If you haven't used the things in it once through the annual cycle the chances are you can do without them. Throw them away. If you are still in two minds about something, ask yourself a few simple questions:

Do I need it?

Does it make me feel good?

Does it feel like me?

Can I realistically expect to use it?

How easy would it be to replace if I were to get rid of it and regret it?

Am I refusing to let go of it because I am clinging on to something from my past which it would be better to let go of?

Storage Space

Once you have cleared away the clutter from your life, you will need to organize your space effectively so that your possessions all have a proper place to live. If you don't already have storage space for everything, go out and buy some affordable units such as concertina files, boxes or drawers. Keep items together which are used for the same purpose so they are easy to find. Make specific spaces for in-between items as well – where do you put the clothes you have worn and plan to wear again? Where do half-read magazines live? If everything has a place then clutter shouldn't accumulate.

This is also a good opportunity to evaluate how well you are using your living space. Could your rooms be better organized? If you generally eat in the kitchen or in front of the television could you use your dining area for something else? Might it be sensible to allocate the largest room to the children and make the living room a toy-free zone for grown-ups? Is there an attic which might be put to better use, or could you clear out the garage and use the space for something else?

As soon as an area is clear, give it a thorough clean. Polish, wipe and hoover every nook and cranny. Clean the bugs and dust-mites out of your carpets and dry-clean the curtains. Open the windows and let fresh air in. You are letting go of your old life and welcoming in the new.

Keeping It Clear

When you have completed your clear-out you should feel quite liberated. The atmosphere in your home will be lighter and less stressful and you may well have gained confidence now that your life is better organized. Bringing a little organization into your home does not just make space, you will find it saves you time as well. The challenge now is to avoid the clutter building up again.

If you have a place for everything and you make the effort to keep everything in its place, clutter shouldn't build up again unless you bring more in. Before introducing anything into your home ask yourself two questions:

Do I need it?
Do I have space for it?

If the answer to either of these is 'no' then **keep it out**!

You might be particularly vulnerable to clutter if you buy things specifically because they are fashionable. Buying this season's colour or design is all very well if you can afford it and if you have enough space. Otherwise, before you bring something in make room for it by throwing something out. There are websites which are specifically designed for auctioning off unwanted goods so there is no need to lose out financially.

Energy Enhancers

Once your home is free of negative clutter you can begin to fill it with positive energy enhancers.

Feng shui

The art of **feng shui** (pronounced 'feng shway') is perhaps the most widely recognized method of creating positive living energy. Unfortunately, this ancient tradition has been rather hijacked by a lunatic fringe in recent years and has received a bad press. In its true form it is a highly complex practice which undoubtedly contains some wisdom. It is concerned with dissolving, deflecting and balancing the negative forces in a space and allowing positive energy to flow in. At its deepest level, feng shui is the interplay between the seen (our surroundings) and the unseen (energy and intention).

Traditional feng shui maintains that the layout of a space will have a profound impact on the energy it instils in people. Walk around your house or garden and consider ways in which the layout might be improved. For example, is the sofa in the sitting room facing towards the television with its back to the door? We sometimes feel more comfortable when we can see who is coming into a room and it may make the room more welcoming to move the furniture around so that it is facing the other way.

29

Light

Did you know that levels of the mood and sleep hormone melatonin are triggered by natural light? If you don't get enough natural light during the day you may be laying yourself open to disturbed sleep, lethargy and depression. When fluorescent strip-lights expire, replace them with full-spectrum light bulbs. These can be obtained in most specialist light shops or large department stores. Full-spectrum bulbs simulate approximately 90% of natural light and are particularly good to have in work spaces.

Beautiful lighting is key to creating a positive environment. Use lamps or candles instead of overhead lights to create an atmosphere of intimacy or relaxation, or fit a dimmer switch to overhead lights. Mirrors add a sense of light and space to any room. A well-placed mirror can make a gloomy room feel light and spacious and reduce the need for extra lighting.

Noise

Noise is audible clutter. The word **noise** is derived from the Latin word 'nausea' meaning sea sickness. There is no doubt that noise is a pervasive pollutant and excessive noise can be insidious. During the summer months many cities become building sites and even the more remote corners of our world are no longer free from the sound of jet engines. Second-hand noise, which is noise created by someone else without our consent, is generally recognized as being more stressful than noise which we generate ourselves. Someone operating a drill or leaf blowing machine is less likely to be stressed by the noise than their neighbours.

We all have some measure of control over the noise in

our immediate environment. Do you always turn the radio or television on when you are alone? If so, is it as much through force of habit as anything? Don't be afraid of silence. It won't hurt you. Music can be both soothing or uplifting, but a few minutes of silent mindfulness each day might be just as beneficial. In the same way, do you walk along busy pavements on your way to work each morning, beset by the roar of traffic? If so, have you considered taking a different route to work, or wearing earplugs? Both of these will reduce your noise stress significantly and make the noise you can't control easier to cope with.

Air

Fresh air is also important. Fresh air contains positive and negative ions – electrically charged particles. Central heating, cigarette smoke and general pollution can cause the air in your house to become charged with too many positive ions. This is believed to contribute to tiredness, headaches, breathing disorders, allergies and depression. If you want to know what having plenty of negative ions in the air feels like, go and stand next to a waterfall – you will be instantly refreshed.

Always sleep with the window open a little, unless you are staying in a polluted environment. You won't feel the cold if you are snuggled up under enough layers, no matter what the weather is like outside. You can charge your environment with negative ions by investing in an ionizer. Some people also like to have a humidifier in their bedroom. This helps to keep moisture at the right level for healthy breathing and your skin benefits too.

A less expensive alternative is to invest in some pot plants. Plants purify the air naturally through the process of photosynthesis. As they absorb light they remove toxic organic pollutants from the air and provide a steady supply of fresh oxygen. You don't need to turn your house into a garden centre; one 12-inch potted plant can clean the air of a medium-sized room.

Colour

Few people are aware of the extent to which colour can alter our mood. Studies have demonstrated that the colour of a room in a school or hospital can affect learning and recovery. Just adding different colours or more colour can considerably alter a room's energy. Red is recognized as being empowering, but it can also be overpowering if used in excess. Soft orange walls or furnishings can be stimulating, warming and relaxing. Yellow is also a warming colour and it can be nurturing and cosy. Blue is often associated with coldness and anxiety but it can be a cleansing and invigorating colour. Like green, it can cool and soothe.

Of course, people respond to different colours subjectively. What is cool and soothing to one person might seem cold and austere to another. Take a few minutes to consider what colours are most appealing to you and why. If green is a colour that enlivens or invigorates you then it may not be the best choice for your bedroom.

Fragrance

You might like to burn aromatherapy oils around the house. It is important that you use the right oils to create the desired mood or effect. Lavender is great for helping you sleep. You can even put a couple of drops of lavender oil on the pillow or relax in a lavender bath – a couple of drops of oil under the running water, no more – before going to bed. As with noise, there are plenty of people who are smell-sensitive so be sure that everyone in the house approves before you light a joss-stick!

You might find as you work through this book that your needs and tastes change. You may want to create an atmosphere which is a little calmer and a little warmer than you had previously enjoyed. Don't rush into creating a new colour scheme or buy a new three-piece suite until you have started to settle into your new self.

Sacred Space

You have cleared out your clutter and turned your home into a positive and nurturing environment. Your last task is to set aside a small area which you can call your own, for instance a meditation mat or chair in the corner of the bedroom that you can retreat to whenever you wish or when you do not want to be disturbed. The simplest thing you can do is to make the bathtub your sacred space for a while each evening. Light some candles and an oil burner in the bathroom or add a few drops of aromatherapy oil to the warm water. Hang a note on the door asking that you are not disturbed and allow yourself time to relax. This is your space and your time to enjoy it.

Clearing away the clutter from your home and finding ways to add a few energy enhancers should considerably improve the atmosphere of your home, but if you ask a child what makes a happy home the answer won't be expensive furniture or a neat lawn. Children respond to love and security and we, as adults, are no different. A happy atmosphere is far more valuable than a well-made bed.

The emotional atmosphere of any space is largely dependent on the people who live or work there. A negative atmosphere caused by resentment, confrontation or abuse will profoundly affect the mood of anyone who enters that environment. If you are at ease with yourself and the world this spirit of serenity and goodwill will carry itself through into your home. The best way to create a positive environment is to create light and happiness within yourself.

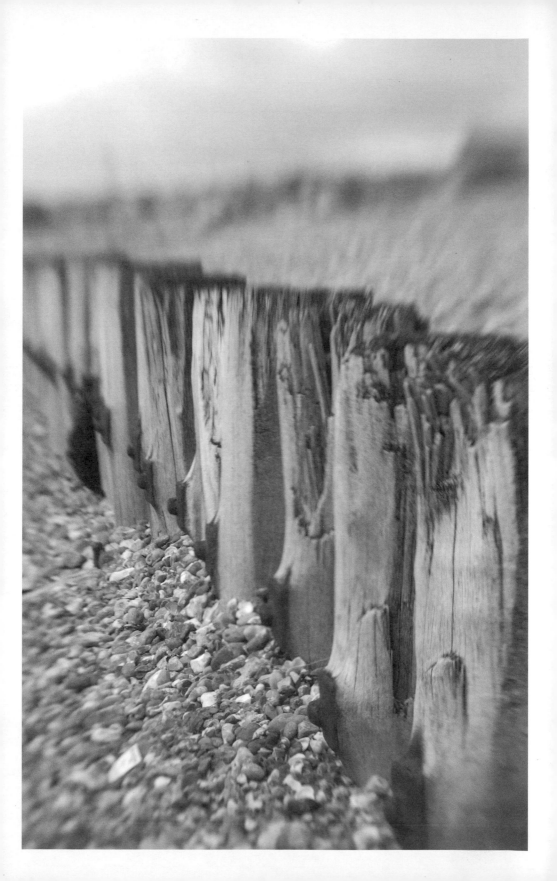

3 | Detoxing Your Finances

Heather: *I've always been pretty good with my finances because my dad was always in debt and I didn't want to make the same mistake. Once you've lived with debt and seen the corrosive effect it can have on people and their lives you will do your utmost to avoid it. When my first marriage ended I took very little money from the divorce, but I had run up some debts. I rolled them into a single loan, took on a number of different jobs to meet my debt repayments, and – gruelling though it sometimes was – I paid it all off. Money can be a major source of anxiety and the best way to overcome this worry is to face it head-on and take control. Once again you need to get organized.*

Ben: *The main reason my television production company collapsed, if I'm being brutally honest, was poor money-management. I seemed to be earning a lot so I started to enjoy myself. I bought a Bentley and refurbished the house. I took my eye off the ball, in other words. After the business collapsed I was left with debts of about £100,000, which wasn't fun, and my creditors weren't interested in sob stories: they just wanted to be paid. Heather encouraged me to face the situation and take* *control. I did so and I have retained that control ever since. Even crippling debts can be manageable. Whether you are wealthy or in debt the chances are your financial situation could be improved. If you are a home-owner, your biggest expense is likely to be the roof over your head, so let's start there.*

Mortgage

If you own your own property the easiest way to save money is often to find a new mortgage. At the time of writing this, by shopping around and cutting 2% off a mortgage of £100,000, it is possible to save about £160 a month. Find out if you are tied into your existing mortgage and whether you are tied into a redemption penalty. If you are free to change your mortgage, don't ask just one bank or building society for their best deal as they will only look at their own products. Head down to the high street and spend a couple of hours examining the market and comparing the different deals on offer. The mortgage industry is cut-throat and there are generally a variety of special deals on offer. It is likely that some of these will improve upon your existing mortgage.

Once you have seen what else is available, ask your existing lender if they will improve your current deal by matching what's out there. They will be keen to hang on to an existing customer and you may be surprised at their readiness to be flexible. Even a small cut in interest can save you a great deal of money over the lifetime of the mortgage.

Utility bills

You could cut the cost of your utilities significantly by switching to a different gas or electricity supplier. With a small amount of effort on your part you could make big savings.

When you change suppliers the pipes and circuits to your home remain the same, all that changes is the cost of the gas or electricity. Switching suppliers should be a smooth process: you take a meter reading and the supplier does the rest.

There are a number of companies on the internet providing free comparison services which can advise you on the most appropriate providers to switch to. Simply type in your post-code and approximate usage and they will do the rest. If the comparison company administers the switch on your behalf – rather than merely advising you on the best option – you might also be able to get cash back. It is always worth enquiring if you are eligible.

When you switch to the cheapest supplier set up a fixed monthly direct debit payment. This could save you up to 10% on your bills, an incentive offered by the supplier because they will be earning interest on any overpayments you make. You can keep overpayments to a minimum by reading your meter at regular intervals. Anything you have overpaid should be refunded to you immediately or at the end of the year.

You don't always have to go to the internet. Your local library is a mine of information, especially if it holds back copies of *Which?* magazine. Ask the librarian to help you find what you are looking for.

Phone bills

The big home phone companies make a lot of noise in their advertising campaigns about who is the cheapest of them all. Unlike the gas and electricity comparison services, the phone comparison services get their commission from the bigger phone companies and therefore tend to point you towards switching to these big companies. You would be much better looking to the numerous smaller, less high-profile, phone companies, as this is where the real price war is going on. An hour or two spent surfing on the internet should give you a variety of options to choose from.

Some of the cheapest (and most obscure) phone providers require you to dial a prefix number (such as 18866 or 1899) before dialling the number you are calling but it is worth it. The savings more than make up for the inconvenience factor, especially as you should be able to have the prefix number as one of the programmable buttons on your phone.

A single phone call may be all it takes to reduce your mobile phone bill. Call your network and tell them that you are considering transferring your account to another company. Nine times out of ten – and occasionally with a little prompting from you: 'I haven't made up my mind for certain yet, but the saving is about 5% and I was wondering if you could match this?' – they will attempt to keep your custom by offering you an equivalent or better package.

Water rates

Thousands of people are paying more than they need to for water. If you are not on a meter, your water rates will be evaluated on the number of bedrooms in your property. If you have fewer people living in your property than you have bedrooms, ask your water supplier to switch you to a water meter. The approximate average unmetered bill in England and Wales for 2005 was £244, while the average metered bill was £209.

The cost of installing a meter will usually be covered by the water company unless they can demonstrate that it is justifiably impractical. If your non-essential water usage is clearly going to be high – if you have a swimming pool, for instance – they will generally fit a meter whether you request it or not. Check with your local supplier.

Once on a meter you can immediately lower your water consumption by placing a brick or a large fizzy drink bottle filled with water in the cistern above your toilet. This will reduce the quantity of water used with each flush. Keep an eye on your metered bills and compare them to the old, unmetered bills. You have the right to switch back within 12 months, or within a month of getting your second metered bill, whichever is later.

Insurance
It is worth checking your household and car insurance costs regularly, especially at the time of renewal. If you simply renew your insurance with the same company year on year you can find that costs have increased without your really being aware of it.

The most obvious way of cutting your household insurance is to reduce the risk of having to make an insurance claim. Fitting approved locks and installing alarm systems can be counterproductive if you are spending more on security than you can ever save on insurance. Schemes such as Neighbourhood Watch, however, can reduce insurance bills and they cost nothing. Another way of making a saving is to increase the excess on your policy (the amount you pay towards any claim you make).

The next thing to do is shop around. You could do this through a broker but, as insurance brokers tend to stick to a small number of companies and throw a consultancy fee of their own into the mix, you can't always guarantee to get the best deal this way. One of the simplest ways to access a large number of companies is to log on to an insurance supermarket website by keying 'insurance supermarket' into a search engine. These will trawl through 50–100 direct sales companies and brokers looking for the best deal. The entire process can be completed in a matter of minutes. Take down the details of the top three companies quoted and visit their individual websites. Put in your information again for a requote as the price may vary with a more detailed enquiry and you may find that you are entitled to further reductions by buying online. Now get on the phone and (you've guessed it) haggle. Leave the cheapest company until last and ask the other two if they will improve upon this quote. Finally, take the best quote to your existing insurer and see if they will beat it. You are about to discover that there is no such thing as a fixed insurance quote!

Credit Cards

The amount you owe on a credit card can get out of hand quicker than you would believe. The trick is to manage credit cards intelligently and never, ever be tempted to bury your head in the sand.

It's not uncommon for people to try to pay off a credit card charging 13% interest by taking out an overdraft at the bank at 18% interest. This is crazy. Either switch bank account (some banks and building societies offer 0% overdrafts for a year to new clients paying in a salary in excess of £6,000–7,000 p/a) or switch the debt on your existing credit card to one with a 0% offer for balance transfers. There are so many cards offering 0% interest on balance transfers that it is possible to switch your borrowings from card to card as each 0% offer runs out and end up paying no interest at all. Watch out for transfer fees, though.

When you switch cards simply tell the new card provider which of your cards you want to transfer a balance from (and how much you want to transfer – you don't have to transfer all of it if you don't want to) and they will do the rest for you. Be careful not to spend on a card after transferring a balance on to it, unless it clearly states 0% interest on purchases as well as transfers, as you could end up paying high interest again.

Shop around for the longest 0% deal available and if you have not paid off your debt at the end of this period switch to another 0% card. This may seem disloyal but it is a service offered and it means that your debts remain interest-free. Be certain to switch cards in plenty of time. You will need to apply for a new 0% card about six weeks before the deadline on the one you have, so don't forget to put it in your diary!

Even with a 0% deal you will still be required to meet a minimum monthly repayment. The best way of ensuring you meet this requirement is to set up a monthly direct debit. You can always top up the repayments to pay the debt off more quickly.

When you have paid off your debt, start using your credit card to your advantage. Some credit cards will even give you money for spending – 1% on everything you buy in some cases – which can add up to quite a tidy sum if you regularly use your credit cards. As long as you pay off your card each month you won't be penalized.

Savings

If your savings account is paying less than the rate of inflation you are 'saving' nothing. If the rate of inflation stands at 10% and your savings account is generating 5% you are losing money, in real terms, at the rate of 5% a year. Interest rates on savings accounts are quoted gross (before tax) but in fact you will need to pay tax on interest earned so you may be earning even less on your savings than you thought. If this is the case, your savings need urgent attention.

Begin by considering your borrowings. The interest your money generates in a savings account is very likely to be less than what it is costing you to borrow money elsewhere. Your first task should be to use your savings to minimize your borrowings.

Next, transfer any remaining savings from your regular savings account to a cash ISA, which is just like a regular savings account but without tax. Regular savings accounts and cash ISAs have a limit on how much you can put in. If you have significant savings put them in an instant access savings account which has no limit.

There is another option available to you if you have savings. 'Saving' means just that, putting money to one side without risk. 'Investing', on the other hand, means taking some risk but the potential returns are higher. Before you put your cash in a savings account it might be worth considering investing instead. The downside, of course, is that there is the possibility that you could lose the lot. Consider your options with caution, but always try to make your money work for you – after all, you worked hard for your money.

Shopping

Online retailers have lower overheads than high street stores and this is generally reflected in their prices. Prices range on the internet every bit as much as they do in the high street and it always pays to shop around but, on the whole, buying anything from airline tickets to shoes can be easier, quicker and less expensive on the internet.

Most goods can be located through a search engine or by calling the retailers themselves and asking for their website address. If you don't want to actually buy off the internet, use it to generate a comparison price list to take to high street retailers and see if they will price-match it. There's no harm in asking!

Shopping robots (otherwise known as 'shopbots') are special websites which scan the internet for the cheapest prices. Kelko and Dealtime are two such sites. You will need to factor in delivery costs, but the cost of delivering several items is often the same as delivering just one. Most shopbots make their income directly from the retailers they list so it is always advisable to try two or three shopbot sites in order to get the greatest possible spread of retailers. This need only take a few minutes and it will be significantly quicker than checking out 100 stores individually.

Travel

It's generally thought that the best way to get a cheap holiday is to rush into a travel agent at the last moment and take anything they have but there are plenty of other ways to holiday inexpensively. For instance, it is now comparatively easy to shop around on the internet for the best no-frills flight and locate an affordable hotel yourself, thereby cutting the travel agent and their fees out of the equation altogether.

Another option, often disregarded, is to book early through a travel agent. If you have a specific destination in mind with defined services, such as facilities for children, then booking your holiday nine or ten months in advance might entitle you to a discount or free trips. A great way of saving money on a holiday is to take your break, if you can, at unfashionable times of the year, especially outside the school summer holidays if you don't have children of school age. The weather and the scenery can be every bit as lovely in June as in August and the queues are likely to be shorter. Many fabulous destinations are hot all year round so you can have your summer break in December.

Try Teletext. Teletext lists the names and phone numbers of holiday companies offering packages to your destination. Make a note of these, make yourself a cup of tea and get your dialling finger out. The prices quoted on Teletext are likely to be significantly cheaper than the brochure price. Find the cheapest quote for your destination then ring one of the other companies listed and ask if they can beat it. Now call another company and ask them if they can improve upon this new quote. Repeat the process three or four times and a holiday with a brochure price of, say, £600 could be yours for £350. Now move your attention from the location specialists to companies whose ads on Teletext state that they will beat any quote. Don't spend more than an hour on this or you will get obsessive, but haggling can be fun and with savings like that it's time well spent.

Of course, if you are feeling brave you can leave it to the

very last minute then approach a travel agent and see what deals they have on offer – and haggle! Last-minute deals on holidays are rarely absolute and, like market traders selling off their fruit and veg on a Saturday evening, they will be keen to offload their remaining stock.

Saving money isn't rocket science. There are plenty of things most of us can do to improve our financial situation. You don't need to believe us, there are some great websites out there with up-to-date information on how to save money, such as www.moneysavingexpert.com. These will give you the most up-to-date deals on mortgage rates, credit card savings and so on. They are a great place to start and a great place to check on regularly.

Finally, whatever your situation you can afford to be charitable. Visit www.thehungersite.com and click on the 'Give Free Food' icon. Simply by clicking on this icon every morning you can ensure that one starving person will receive a meal that day. Even giving to charity can be done without spending anything!

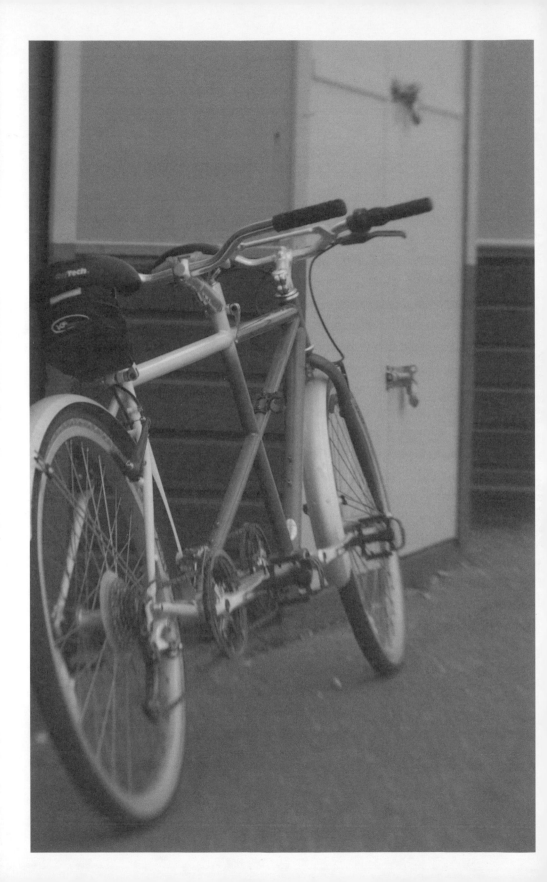

4 | Looking Great

Heather: *When I lived in a caravan I had a bucket instead of a toilet and things were pretty basic, but I still made sure I put my make-up on every morning. And I would do it for me, for my own sense of self-esteem, rather than for the benefit of people I met. When I was feeling low I would splash out 99p on a pot of nail varnish or a nail file. There's a great phrase I heard recently, 'Fake it to make it.' It's amazing what good taking care of yourself can do for your morale.*

Ben: *Losing interest in your appearance is generally recognized as an early sign of depression or low self-esteem and it's often self-generating. If you begin to let yourself go your morale will soon slump. Years ago, when I was working as a road sweeper in London, I loved to put on a suit and tie to go to the theatre and sit in the balcony. Just wearing a suit changed my bearing and it gave a real boost to my self-esteem. People react far more positively towards you if you take care of yourself.*

Heather: *I do think it's a pity that the way you look is quite so important. You are judged on it, immediately, rather than on what really matters – your spirit. Mind you, this can play to your* *advantage. I do quite a lot of public speaking and people respond very differently to me when I'm wearing a smart suit. Perhaps they think I'm more intelligent when I'm smartly dressed – they certainly behave and speak in ways which suggest this! Only Richard Branson can get away with wearing a fluffy jumper and jeans at a corporate meeting. I'm aware that your clothes can be a useful tool in terms of gaining the confidence of others and boosting your self-esteem. After all, who can fail to feel good about themselves if they know they look great?*

Walk down the street with your shoulders hunched and your head hanging low, looking at the pavement as you drag your feet. Be mindful of how this makes you feel. Now repeat the exercise but this time with your shoulders back, your chin up and your head held high. You cannot help feeling more positive if you assume the posture of an upbeat person. This can be a very useful trick when you're feeling a bit under the weather. Even when you are alone and unobserved by others, one of the most effective ways of increasing your confidence can be to assume the appearance of confidence.

Non-Verbal Communication

Around 70% of human communication is non-verbal. When you meet someone you may not be consciously aware of the extent to which you 'judge' them on the basis of their body language. Their shoulders are a little hunched: perhaps they don't want to be noticed and they lack confidence? They are not meeting your gaze: maybe they are hiding something?

They are staring you down and not blinking: you don't like them, they strike you as being a little too aggressive.

Your body sends out a thousand signals with every meeting, every conversation, and the unconscious mind of the observer cannot help but be influenced by these sub-liminal messages, often interpreted as gut feelings: 'There's just something about her...' The language of the human body is universal. A slouched stance, downcast eyes, a furrowed brow, clenched teeth, all of these say something very clear about you, even when you remain silent.

But, like any language, this can be mastered. The rules are fairly simple. Be genuine, open and reasonably confident and you can't go wrong. A fake smile or brash overconfidence can be counterproductive. If you feel good about yourself, on the other hand, this message will come across to everyone.

Look After Your Skin

The first thing to suffer when you stop looking after yourself is the condition of your skin. Have you been eating badly? Drinking too much? Your skin will shout about it to the world.

Heather: *Nowadays, it takes me just a few minutes to get ready before I go out. Even when I've got a toddler around my feet I still set aside five to ten minutes to care for my appearance. If I have organized my time properly, I set aside half an hour each morning to do my routine: I get up, exfoliate my face, followed by a shower where I wash my hair. All year round I use a strong sun protection cream on my chest and face – SPF 60. I apply a tinted moisturizer, a bit of mascara, some light lippy, and that's that.*

There are still some days when I allow myself to look pretty

51

scruffy. That's when the paparazzi break cover from the bushes and get their shot. But we've all got to have time out every now and again, and I'm only human. Mind you, because I look so scruffy in some of the photos, people have occasionally come up to me in the street and said, 'You look quite smart in real life!' I think it's supposed to be a compliment!

Human skin needs two basic things in order to look healthy: hydrogen and oxygen. For many people, bad skin is a result of lifestyle choices. By keeping out of direct sunlight, eating a good diet, avoiding cow's milk as it has been heavily linked with acne, avoiding stress, getting enough sleep, doing simple breathing exercises and drinking plenty of water, your skin will remain happy and healthy – all of your skin, not just your face.

Another thing that affects the quality of your skin is the amount of exercise you take. When you begin to exercise regularly fatty tissue dies away and muscle mass increases, which stretches your skin tighter. This will be particularly evident on your upper arms and shoulders, and on your buttocks and thighs. After just a few weeks your skin should begin to feel younger, smoother and more supple.

Whatever the temptation, the last thing you should do is overexpose your skin to the sun. Too much sun irreversibly ages the skin on your face and body.

Heather: *As a teenager I was constantly on sunbeds, so much so that eventually I ended up with pigmentation patches on my face. It wasn't until I was in my 20s that I learnt about skin cancer. I haven't sunbathed for 15 years. I prefer to keep out of the sun and wear a fake tan. There's no tan in the world which is* *so wonderful that it couldn't have come out of a bottle. Most high street chemists have a selection of fake tans which look every bit as good as the real thing; the days when bottled tans had a rather sinister orange glow to them are, thankfully, in the past! Most people look better with some colour.*

If you have overdone it, one of the best ways to minimize the effects of sun damage, hyper-pigmentation, acne, premature signs of ageing, and many more skin conditions, is a glycolic or salicylic acid face peel. Consult a dermatologist or skin care professional for advice on what is best for your particular skin.

Cellulite

Women store fat six times more easily in their lower body than the upper, and over 90% of women say that they suffer from cellulite. Its primary causes are believed to be poor diet (particularly junk food, additives and pesticide residues), hormone imbalance (meaning that taking the Pill and HRT can both contribute to cellulite), poor digestion and stress. Poor digestion is often due to lack of water, fresh fruit and vegetables. Begin by cutting out processed, packaged or ready-prepared foods and switch to a more healthy diet. Eat plenty of protein and cut down on fatty or sugary foods which might try to take up permanent residence on your thighs as cellulite. Cut down on dairy products and drink plenty of pure or filtered water. Supplement your diet with a good multi-vitamin/mineral every day.

Exercise is another key factor in overcoming cellulite, particularly stretching and toning activities such as swimming, yoga or dancing.

As a last resort you may want to try liposuction (a process whereby fat is sucked from the body in a syringe) but the results for this condition are not always convincing. Surgery of this sort can be both expensive and risky and, if you don't keep up a healthy lifestyle, the cellulite will return.

Look After Your Smile

Nothing beats a beautiful smile for lighting up a face. The rules for caring for your teeth are simple and we all know them. Brush twice a day, once after rising and once before bed. If your teeth are healthy, an electric toothbrush is more effective than a standard brush, in the same way that an electric floor polisher can do a better job than polishing the floor by hand. Be sure to brush the insides of your teeth, especially towards the front, as this is where saliva is produced and with saliva comes plaque-forming minerals. Floss your teeth daily to help prevent gum disease, preferably using flat, wide floss because it doesn't shred so easily.

Keep an eye on what you consume. The potential damage done by eating too many sweets or foods high in sugar has been well-documented. Red wine, tea and coffee stain the teeth, although toothpastes are now available which are formulated to remove such stains. Citrus fruits such as orange or grapefruit create an acid environment in your mouth which can lead to decay so it's best to clean your teeth after eating them or drinking their juices. Smoking stains your teeth, makes your breath smell and contributes to gum shrinkage and increased risk of infection.

Millions of bacteria accumulate on your tongue every day, which looks unsightly and can lead to bad breath. Brush your tongue when you brush your teeth, and scrape your tongue with a tongue-scraper at least once a week.

Go to your dentist for a check-up once a year and see your dental hygienist every six months or so to have plaque and surface stains removed. If you don't like your teeth the way they are, don't be afraid to discuss your dislikes with your dentist. A lot of high street dentists now offer bleaching treatments and other cosmetic dentistry and will be happy to talk over all the options with you.

Fighting the Biomarkers

No part of your body is much older than a year. Every three months your skeleton is renewed. Every six weeks your liver renews itself. Even your skin, one of the most obvious indicators of ageing, renews its cells entirely every month. So what does 'ageing' mean and why do we fear it?

Your age is determined by your body's 'biomarkers' – measurable markers of age which include such factors as skin condition, blood pressure, flexibility, muscle mass and body posture. Yet it's not just the passing years which cause changes in your biomarkers. Stress, a poor diet and lack of exercise all contribute. If you fail to look after yourself your 'biological age' will be greater than your 'chronological age'. You will look older than your years, in other words. Your skin will wrinkle, you may become less flexible, your blood pressure could rise.

Studies suggest that exercising – and in particular strength training – is the best way to improve measurable markers of ageing such as fat composition, skin elasticity, body strength, coordination and reflexes. When you take up exercise in adult life for the first few months you will actually seem to be growing younger as your muscles tighten up, your posture improves and energy levels increase. In the long-term, regular exercise can slow down the rate of ageing.

Regular exercise also keeps your blood pressure under control, which in turn helps protect you from developing kidney disease, heart disease and strokes. Regular activity also lowers blood glucose levels, which can help prevent the onset of diabetes.

The body's metabolic rate decreases every ten years or so which means that by the end of each decade your body is burning 100 fewer calories each day on average than it did at the beginning of each decade. These extra calories tend to pile on the inches. Exercise helps to slow down this metabolic slide and encourages your metabolism to be more efficient. Regular exercise enables you to burn more calories (even when you are resting), improves your complexion and puts a sparkle in your eyes. We will be discussing exercise in more detail in a later chapter.

Posture is another important biomarker. Few things betray old age more clearly than the way someone moves and carries themselves. But, whereas many in the medical profession look on pain and stiffness as natural side-effects of old age, there is increasing evidence to suggest that this need not necessarily be so. Regular practitioners of Pilates, the Alexander Technique and yoga tend to retain good posture right into old age, which suggests that far from being an inevitable side effect of the ageing process, poor posture can be avoided.

And your posture can have a direct bearing on your mood. If you slump your shoulders the volume of your chest cavity is reduced causing shallow breathing which can have a negative effect on your sense of well-being. When you are sitting or standing, imagine being suspended from a piano wire attached to the top of your head. Your strength should emanate from your spine, rather than from the muscles of your body. Placing undue pressure on your muscles hour after hour will inevitably deplete your energy levels. For an immediate spine and posture straightener, when you sit down, pull your butt cheeks out from under you until you can feel that you are sitting on your 'sit bones'. Voilà!

Be Graceful

Take reasonable precautions to arrest the signs of ageing, but do so with grace. It is one thing to do what we can to look youthful but it's quite another to overdo it! A woman in late middle age with bleached blonde hair and caked make-up can lack dignity, just as can a man who sweeps a few strands of hair over a bald patch or someone who wears an obvious toupee.

We all grow old in time but it is possible to look great well into old age if you exude positive energy and look after yourself. Ultimately, all the words we tend to associate with ageing – slow, weak, doddering, stooped, saggy – need not apply to you if you care for yourself properly. Don't put all your faith in a boob job, liposuction, a face lift, hair transplant, or getting waxed or plucked or tweaked. These are good for morale but they will only give you a short-term boost. If you're not confident and happy on the inside, they won't make a jot of difference in the long-run. The secret to beating the ageing process is **feeling** great – being fit and healthy.

Heather: *Personally, I believe that a person's true beauty comes from within. And I mean that literally, not as some flaky New Age statement. There is far more to attractiveness than physique, the clothes you wear or your hairstyle. What we generally find attractive in other people is their spirit as it shines through in their confidence, their bright eyes, the way they talk and how they carry themselves. I was interested to read that at Harvard Medical School it was discovered that people with high self-esteem tend to be more upbeat and happy, and that these outward exhibitions of their inner confidence make other people react positively to them, which in turn increases their self-esteem. If you make the effort to look after yourself, body and soul, you will inevitably feel great and an unavoidable consequence of feeling great is looking great. I'll leave you with some wonderful beauty tips from one of Audrey Hepburn's favourite poems that she quoted:*

For lovely lips, speak words of kindness.
For lovely eyes, seek out the good in people.
For a slim figure, share your food with the hungry.
For beautiful hair, let a child run his or her fingers
    through it once a day.
For poise, walk with the knowledge you'll never walk
    alone.
People, even more than things, have to be restored,
    renewed, revived, reclaimed, and redeemed; never
    throw out anybody.
As you grow older, you will discover that you have two
    hands, one for helping yourself, the other for helping
    others.
The beauty of a woman is not the clothes she wears, the

figure that she carries, or the way she combs her hair.

The beauty of a woman must be seen in her eyes, because that is the doorway to the heart, the place where love resides.

True beauty in a woman is reflected in her soul. It is the caring that she lovingly gives and the passion that she shows.

And the beauty of a woman with passing years only grows.

The second essential key to a lifetime of well-being:

EMOTIONAL EQUILIBRIUM

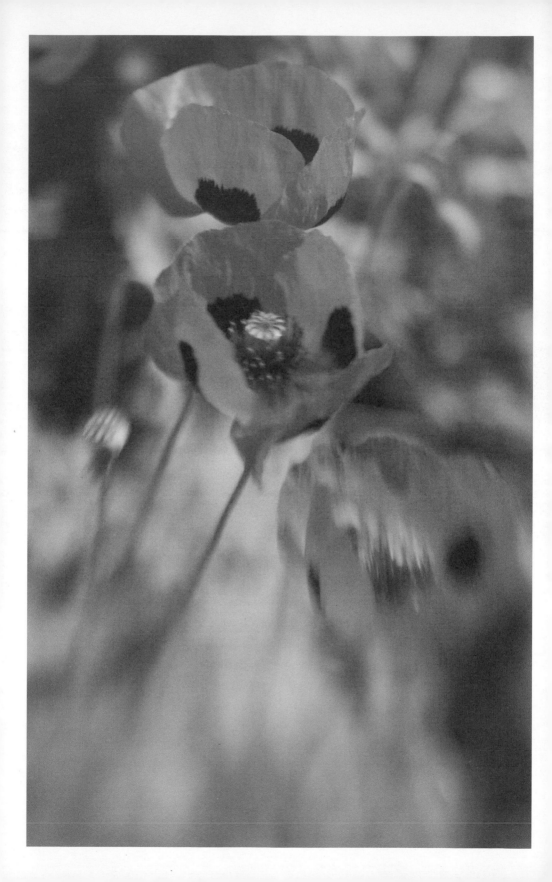

5 | Raising Self-Esteem

Heather: *I've been in the public eye for some years, ever since I lost my leg, but I had no problems with my relationship with the media until I got married. The press made me out to be a gold-digger and I decided to keep my mouth shut and say nothing. Looking back, I think that was a mistake. That period turned out to be the darkest and most difficult in my life – worse even than losing my leg. Celebrity is a curious animal and too much praise, like too much criticism, can be damaging. Nowadays I don't take myself too seriously and I try to take everything with a pinch of salt. The experience did, though, teach me a thing or two about the importance of self-esteem.*

Ben: *I remember reading a piece in one of the British tabloids and thinking that the person they were talking about bore no resemblance to the Heather I have known all these years.*

I do think a lot of people empathized with her even when the situation was at its worst. Anyone who has been at the centre of gossip, or been through a divorce, for instance, knows how easily people make judgements about someone based on half-truths and hearsay. If you are on the receiving end the sense of injustice can be profound and it can completely shatter your sense of

63

self-worth. Through knowing Heather, I have learnt to be some-what distant – and sceptical – when I read about a personality in a newspaper or hear someone being talked about when they are not there to answer back. In the following chapters we will be exploring equilibrium and self-esteem issues. In my experience as a counsellor, I have discovered that taking the time to address your emotional health is an essential key to life balance and well-being.

Heather: *I have a group of close friends I love dearly and who know me well. One thing they share in common is an aversion to bad-mouthing people. I used to enjoy a bit of gossip, the same as the next person, but now I realize how profoundly unfair and damaging this can be.*

Most of us muddle through life feeling okay-ish about ourselves and our lives. Even if you are fairly happy and successful in your personal and professional life, everyone has the potential for higher self-esteem. We could all do with a little extra confidence from time to time. Confidence is largely self-generating: people with high self-esteem tend to find it easier to realize their ambitions than those with low self-esteem and their confidence rises with each successful challenge. People react positively towards those with high self-esteem, helping to further boost their confidence. When your self-esteem is high you feel more optimistic about your ability to succeed in your objectives and your energy levels rise to meet them. As you meet your objectives your happiness and self-belief increase. This reinforces your core belief that you are a strong and valuable individual, a belief which feeds your actions and motivates you into further action. The same rules apply to low self-esteem: the lower your confidence levels, the less likely you are to be a high achiever either personally or professionally and life becomes an ever-decreasing circle of low self-worth.

Whereas low self-esteem can permeate almost every aspect of your life, leading to all sorts of physical, emotional and lifestyle difficulties, there can be no denying that the effects of high self-esteem can be very pleasurable. Because of this, people with high self-esteem often devote a significant amount of their energies to increasing their confidence levels. This is, after all, an area of their lives which they have come to associate with feeling good.

Such people are the exception. The truth is that very few of us dedicate much energy to improving our self-worth. This is due, in part, to the fact that very few of us realize the extent to which low self-esteem can affect our health, wealth and relationships. How we feel about ourselves is perhaps the single most pervasive element in our lives, and yet very few people give it a second thought.

Self-Esteem Sappers

All of us have habits, many of them deeply ingrained, which erode our self-esteem. We eat too much, we handle money badly, we are always late, we are disorganized and untidy. Begin by identifying your self-esteem sappers. For the next week, whenever something presents itself that makes you feel less than good about yourself, make a note of it in your notebook. You may be surprised by some of the things you write down. Perhaps you were aware that the grotty paintwork on your front door distressed you a little, but you hadn't realized that it damaged your self-esteem. Crashing out in front of the TV every night or going to bed late might also sap your self-esteem. Also make a note of the things that make you feel anxious or resentful – both are outward expressions of low self-esteem. Perhaps a work colleague tests your patience, but could it be because they make you feel undervalued and insignificant? Identify as many esteem sappers as you can.

Most of us carry around deeply held but largely un-conscious beliefs about ourselves. Things like, 'I am not very attractive,' 'I'm a bit clumsy,' or 'I'm not a very good parent/lover/friend.' Explore some of your own self-beliefs by sitting down with your notebook and allowing some time for free expression: 'I'm basically an okay person, but ...' Nobody is going to see this except you so allow anything to come through, however bizarre or unexpected. This free expression stream of consciousness has been compared with taking a pen for a walk. It can be a highly effective means of uncover-ing some deeply held beliefs about yourself.

Consider the validity of these deeply held beliefs. Human 'mind talk' can be notoriously deceptive so really question these convictions. Put them on the spot and consider which of them, if any, stand up to scrutiny. A great deal of what we tell ourselves about ourselves is based upon misinformation and misunderstanding. This is a good place to put some of these grosser misconceptions to bed. Strike out the ones that are nonsense and add any that are left to your list of esteem sappers.

Prioritize

Now look at your list and prioritize it into significant esteem sappers, medium sappers and mild sappers. The scruffy front door might be a mild sapper whereas you can see that going to bed late significantly affects your self-esteem as it makes you consistently late for work and has a knock-on effect right through the day. Carefully consider each sapper to make sure you are taking into account its knock-on effects. For instance, it may be that you have identified being over-weight as an esteem sapper. Several other sappers on your list such as, 'I don't take care over my appearance,' 'I eat too much junk food,' or, 'I don't take enough exercise,' are a knock-on effect of being overweight. Group them all together on your list.

Identify the things that you can easily do something about – repainting your front door for example, or going to bed earlier. Now take a look at the other things on your list.

Compensate

One of the keys to getting rid of esteem sappers is to identify their compensatory features. Sometimes this is easy: 'I have thin hair, but my eyes are nice.' At other times less so: 'I am a little overweight, but I'm curvy/sexy/being myself.' Compensatory characteristics might be things which you hadn't previously thought of and they often only emerge when you really consider what the upside of a particular problem might be: 'I'm shy with adults but this is possibly why I feel so at ease with children.'

If you look carefully enough through your list the answers

will generally come. If not, focus your attention upon looking for potential compensations: 'Okay, so I'm perhaps a little bossy, but if I handle this properly it could mature into effective leadership.' Every esteem sapper will have either a compensatory feature or the potential for one, if you look hard enough! Write a compensatory feature for each esteem sapper on your list.

It may be that instead of trying to **overcome** some of these sappers, a degree of **acceptance** is preferable – you might be better off accepting your weight rather than attempting to fight it: 'My mother was quite large, I suppose I'm pre-disposed to being on the large side. This is me and I'm fine just as I am. Real women have curves!' This process may take a little time and your self-acceptance is likely to be grudging at first but the consequences of this type of mind-shift can be significant. Instead of being ashamed of yourself you are likely to find you are taking a little more care of your appearance. After a while the focus of your eating might shift away from dieting towards eating for health and vitality. Perhaps you take up exercise, again the focus being on wanting to **feel** good rather than merely **looking** good. Our society tends to measure success by outward appearance rather than on an inner sense of security and serenity – a case of collective deceptive mind talk! Become a free spirit and break the mould. Don't allow yourself to worry about what other people think about you. Be yourself, do your own thing, and others will fit themselves around you. If they don't, you might want to consider the possibility that you are better off without them in your life for a while.

Visualize

Create a clear picture in your mind of the sort of person you would **like** to be. Close your eyes and take a few deep breaths. Envisage the appearance, the mannerisms, the facial expression of the 'ideal you'. See yourself in a location you aspire to – sitting behind the boss's desk, or cuddled up at home with a loved one. Consider the attributes you would like to have. Do you consider yourself to be disorganized? Perhaps your alter-ego is highly efficient and organized. Do you lack confidence? Imagine someone else entering the scene and how you would like to respond towards them. Calm and out-going, perhaps, where normally you would be aggressive or shy? Keep it in the realms of possibility (resist the temptation to turn the clock back ten years) and focus on making this what you would realistically like to achieve. Try to lose yourself in this fantasy for a few minutes. You should now have a clearer idea of some of the attributes you aspire to and the characteristics or aspects of your life you feel you could most benefit from losing. It is now time to address your esteem sappers and eliminate each in turn.

Getting Started

You might want to team up with an ally to tackle certain sappers, for example by taking up exercise with a friend or joining a self-help group. Letting go of the security of a long-held habit or belief about yourself can be unsettling or even frightening and it can be helpful to have the support of another person who shares your objective. Don't be surprised if your new-found interest in exercise has given rise to an increased appetite for sex, sweets or shopping. Some of these impulses may take their toll on your health or your bank balance. Don't lose sight of what it is you are trying to achieve.

An unexpected and surprising impediment to overcoming your esteem sappers can be the attitudes of friends and family. Occasionally they might try to undermine you because they don't want to see you succeeding where they have failed. Others might not see your long-term objectives and witness only your temporary discomfort, which they try to stop because they deem it is bad for you. Don't allow yourself to succumb to their honeyed words! Generally, if you explain what it is you are trying to achieve, people will be encouraging and supportive. If you find someone sapping the lifeblood from you – whatever their motive – you might want to distance yourself from them for a while.

Above all, **think positive**! An affirmation is a positive statement which we repeat regularly to ourselves, such as, 'I enjoy my life,' or 'I am good at my job.' You have created a picture of the sort of person you would like to be and the objectives you would like to fulfil. Create an affirmation you can repeat to yourself whenever you have a quiet moment: 'I feel good about myself and I have the love and respect of others. I can achieve anything I set my mind to.' Write it down in your notebook so that you don't forget it, and repeat it daily. Over time a regularly repeated affirmation can have a surprisingly positive effect.

Reaching Out

Another low effort, high yield way to feel better about yourself is being pleasant to people in your community. The benefits of an improved diet and lifestyle might take a while to make themselves felt, but the response to a smile is immediate. Be pleasant to shop assistants, cab drivers, whoever crosses your path. Make an effort to find out and use people's names. Be friendly and polite on the phone, with strangers as well as with friends. Say 'thank you' to people wherever appropriate, whether to traffic as you cross a road or to other drivers who give way. It is remarkable how many people fail to do this. You might already have made this a way of life, but if not give it a try for a single day and notice what a difference it makes. Taking the time out to say 'hello' and have a brief chat at the checkout or in the street is hard at first but it soon becomes second nature. Most of us lead busy, active lives and it's tempting to get each job done and dispense with all but the necessary pleasantries. Being friendly needn't take up any time – making eye contact or exchanging smiles as you pass someone on the street doesn't take a moment out of your schedule. Be utterly reckless as you spread a little light and happiness around you and watch it come straight back at you. You cannot fail to feel good about yourself if you adopt this attitude.

Dealing With Negativity

There are some fairly simple tricks you can use if you catch yourself being downcast or negative. The first of these is 'reframing'. Speech is one of the clearest indications of negativity and low self-esteem. If you find yourself speaking in terms which are essentially negative, such as 'I'm okay, I suppose – not great,' get into the habit of speaking in more positive terms. Even seemingly negative messages can be delivered in a positive way. 'I'm afraid I can't come to your party, I can only come for a quick drink in the pub beforehand,' becomes, 'I'm really looking forward to joining you in the pub after work. Even if I can't come to the party afterwards, it'll be fun having a drink together.'

'Anchoring' is another useful technique if you find yourself in a position where your confidence might be under threat. Close your eyes, take a few deep breaths, and picture the sights and sounds of an incident when you felt your self-esteem was particularly strong. Think about a task you successfully undertook which might otherwise have daunted you – you stood up to someone, perhaps, or you handled a difficult situation with ease. Remember exactly how you felt. As you picture the scene, make a clear association in your mind with an action (such as pinching your earlobe or pressing your thumb and forefinger together) or an object (such as a bracelet). Repeat this process several times. The next time you are in a challenging situation you can refer to your anchor by glancing at your bracelet or performing your action. Your confidence will rise to help you meet the challenge. We have all seen the countless sportsmen and women who have preferred numbers, favourite colours or particular rituals. This is exactly the same thing. Whoever you are, whatever the occasion, anchoring can be an extremely effective means of boosting confidence.

High self-esteem leads to an increased awareness of others. People who are secure and settled within themselves begin to turn their attention elsewhere. It is little wonder, therefore, that we tend to warm more readily to individuals with high self-esteem. Studies have shown that confidence is a key ingredient in sexual attraction and it can be a significant factor when it comes to promotion at work. Nobody feels inclined to trust their heart or their business to someone who doesn't even trust themselves.

As you raise your own self-esteem remember that truly confident people make the people around them feel at ease, upbeat and stimulated. They are assertive without being bullish and they are likely to stand up for their rights and the rights of others. Remember to bring out the best in the people around you. Be confident enough within yourself not to be threatened by the success of others. Be full of life. These are the pleasures of high self-esteem.

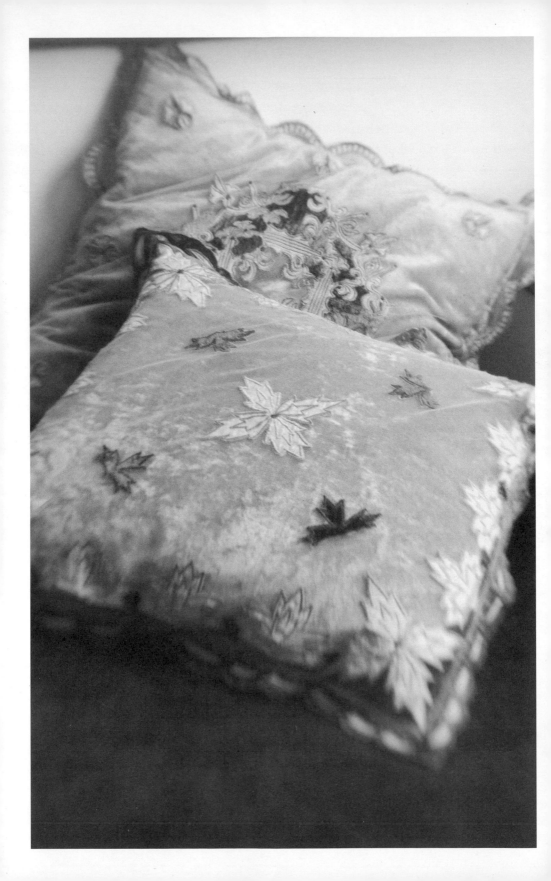

6 | Emotional Detox

Heather: *In our society material accumulation counts for a great deal more than emotional success. As a result very few people take as much care of themselves as they do their possessions. If you tell your friends you are spending the afternoon clearing out the inside of your car they might mumble something about wanting to do the same with theirs, too, if only they had more time. If you tell them that you are spending a few days detoxing your body they might tease you but they will know why you would want to do it. Try explaining to them that you are spending the weekend detoxing your mind and they are likely to be entirely nonplussed. Yet emotional clutter acts as a wall between ourselves and others, and between ourselves and ourselves. We all need to keep on top of our emotional clutter, and it's an ongoing process.*

Ben: *Having undertaken the emotional detox process myself, in the most fearless and thorough way I could muster, I can honestly say that it has been a life-changing experience. It is only by clearing away the emotional blockages of the past that we can experience lasting peace of mind and happiness.*

Life Balance

Welcome to the most rewarding, exciting and (dare I say it) the most challenging section of Life Balance*!*

It is difficult to appreciate the extent to which negative emotions drain us of our health, our self-esteem and our potential. Many people, particularly the British, prefer to keep a stiff upper lip. This is not only detrimental to our emotional well-being and happiness, it can affect physical health, too. Anger, fear and resentment don't simply disappear if you ignore them, they burrow into the unconscious mind where they can remain for years, even decades.

Think back to when you were 13 years old. Your boyfriend has just ditched you and is now seeing that red-headed girl in your class. You felt terrible at the time but you have long since got over it. Right? Wrong. It may be that you no longer have any **conscious** feelings of rejection, hurt or resentment towards either the redhead or your ex, but research has demonstrated that any trauma such as this will be retained in the unconscious mind for years to come.

In other words, that break-up from long ago may still have a hold over you. This might range in influence from the seemingly insignificant (perhaps you have built up a mild distrust of red-headed women) to the more significant, such as a long-lasting fear of emotional intimacy.

The fact is that our experiences can control our subsequent behaviour patterns. They make us who we are, subtly influencing our every move. To a greater or lesser extent we are all influenced by feelings of separation, guilt and fear, built up over a lifetime.

The focus of this chapter is on overcoming the main

obstacles to emotional equilibrium, obstacles such as rejection, low self-esteem and resentment. It is not an easy process and it requires some level of commitment and raw guts from you but once you have done it you will never look back.

The Detox Process

Cast your mind back as far back into your childhood as you can go. Start a fresh page in your notebook and write down the name of anyone who brings up a negative emotion in you, whether it is fear, resentment or anxiety. Write something next to the name to jog your memory when you read the list later, for example:

Uncle Jack	He was a bully, he hit me
John, Infant School	Called me names
Mrs Thomas, my teacher	Ignored me, favoured Jane in my class

Carry the process through to the present day. No matter how small or petty your negative emotion may seem at first, if it occurs to you it must have some significance so set it down on paper:

Traffic warden	Clamped my car
Mrs Jones next door	Often rude to her husband, shouts at him
My children	Not always appreciative of me

Your list should include people, places and things:

Life Balance

ATM machine on high street	Frequently broken
Local car mechanic	Overcharged me

And it should include not just your resentments, but also your fears and disappointments:

Area Manager	Passed me over for promotion
Flying	I hate it!

Also write down the names of all the people you feel you may have harmed – including yourself:

Grandma	I wasn't there for her when she needed me
Me	I let myself down, failed stage school audition

We have all heard the phrases 'I don't believe in raking up the past,' or, 'Let bygones be bygones.' These are admirable sentiments but they completely miss the point. Most emotional clutter lurks in the unconscious mind and few people realize how much it influences them. This isn't rocket science. If you imagine a vat of water with a dead cat in it, the water will be poisoned for as long as the cat lies there. The same is true of your mind. It is only by drawing your negative emotions to the surface that it will be possible to get rid of them. Take a full and frank look at your life – not in self-hate or castigation but with love and compassion. Root out guilt, low self-esteem, fear and resentment wherever you can find them. This is the first step towards dumping negative feelings and moving on.

Your list should end up being several pages long. Most people have a hundred entries or more on their lists. If you don't think you have anything like as much as that to write down it may be that you are not being completely honest with yourself. This is, after all, an emotional stocktake of your **entire** lifetime.

Honesty is crucial to the process. Write down everything that seems significant, no matter how personal it may be. As a rule, the more upsetting, painful or cringe-making the entry, the more important it is that you include it for the greater impact it is likely to have on your emotional welfare. Don't leave out vital details or bend the truth, not even a little! Just tell it as it is and you can't go wrong.

Most people take days, sometimes weeks, to complete their inventories, working on them for half an hour here or an evening there. You will find that long buried feelings of anger and guilt resurface during this process so try not to let it drag on for too long.

Your Positive Attributes

Your completed inventory will be fairly one-sided. Here, in black and white, are all your fears, resentments and regrets. Yet we are controlled by our hopes as much as our fears, by our positive attributes as much as our negative characteristics. Set aside time to ask yourself the following questions:

What things about my personality do I like?
What achievements am I most proud of?

Also ask yourself:

If I were a car, what type of car would I be?
If I were a colour, what colour would I be?
What sort of animal would I be and why?

This is a useful way of revealing attributes which your unconscious mind believes you have: 'I would be a small, sporty car – quite nippy and fun. I would be light blue, cool and refreshing. I would be a squirrel because I've got plenty of initiative.' Ask two or three friends these same questions if you dare. You may be pleasantly surprised by their descriptions of you!

The Clearing Process

This book contains a number of suggestions which require you to stretch your comfort-zone. Detoxing your emotions is no exception. It is not enough to merely complete your list, nor to tuck it away in a box somewhere and move on. You will need to talk it through with someone else.

The person you choose can be a trained counsellor, a trusted friend or a spiritual guide. It can be almost anyone as long as they are discreet and kind and they are willing to share their time with you. Be sensible – don't sit down with your partner or a close friend if you will be telling them things they might find upsetting. This is not an opportunity for you to dump on others irrespective of their feelings.

Set aside sufficient time to discuss each episode on your list in turn with your sharing partner. You may want to complete this over the course of a single weekend or spread it out over several evenings. Create a quiet, comfortable space where you will not be overheard and set to it.

If you are the person who is doing the listening, bear in mind that this clearing process can be draining for both of you. Assure the speaker that your conversation is in total confidence, then your role is to listen. If necessary move things along from time to time, this isn't an opportunity for them to wallow in self-pity or resentment. The idea is that they share their concerns whilst you acknowledge what they have shared. Clearly acknowledging their hurt or anxiety is an important part of the process, then allow them to let go of it and move on to the next item. Don't hurry them un-necessarily. They may have been carrying around some of the things they will be sharing with you for several years. Properly handled, this should be a once-in-a-lifetime exercise for them and it is important that each item on their inventory is given adequate time and attention. You may want to briefly share similar experiences of your own if you feel it will help them to feel more comfortable.

As the speaker works through the items on their list, missing nothing, wounds of many years begin to heal. This is a very powerful process and one which is likely to have a long-term effect on their sense of well-being and happiness. They have made significant inroads into letting go of the more negative and emotionally draining episodes from their past. They might be left with one or two outstanding resent-ments. We will be dealing with these in a moment.

Sharing Your Feelings

Many of us are afraid of telling people who we are. We don't believe it's okay to be ourselves. This belief is often fed by repressed emotions such as low self-esteem, fear or guilt. If you don't want to share your inventory with another person this may be an example of your emotional clutter taking a hold of your responses.

The process of sharing your feelings with another person as a means of letting go is ancient. In many cultures and religious traditions this practice is seen as a touchstone of spiritual progress. Another way of looking at it is to say that negative emotions such as fear or resentment clutter up the pipeline which connects us to other people and to our higher selves, and it is only by getting the plumbers in to clear the blockage that we really open ourselves up. There are times when all of us could do with a little extra support to back up our own resources, no matter how independent we may be. When we're truly honest with another person it overcomes any sense of separateness that we may feel and confirms that we have started being truly honest with ourselves. We don't have to hide any longer.

If you are really not prepared to take this step, don't be entirely disheartened. Just writing it all down can be very cathartic and this is better than nothing. But taking the plunge and sharing your inventory with another person is undoubtedly worth the effort. For many people the feeling of lightness and happiness that ensues from the process is the first concrete affirmation that they have, in fact, been weighed down by emotional baggage. We become so used to lugging it around with us that we don't even realize it's there. The feeling of finally letting go can be wonderful.

Resentment

Resentments are often the most difficult part of the emotional clutter to shift. The word **resentment** stems from the root words meaning 'to feel again' or 'to re-experience' and it is in the nature of a resentment that we can relive it, consciously or unconsciously, for years on end. Just talking it through with a friend sometimes isn't enough. This may be because – and this comes as a surprise to many people – you don't actually **want** to be rid of your resentments.

Clinical psychologist K. Bradford Brown, Ph.D., observed that every resentment has a **cause**, a **payoff** and a **cost**. You have recorded the causes of your resentments in your inventory. What are their payoffs?

Payoff
Your Area Manager passed you over for promotion and you feel justified in your anger towards him. This seems simple enough but are you being entirely honest with yourself? Perhaps they passed you over because there was someone else who was better qualified than you or because another candidate worked harder. In other words, you were unconsciously aware that your Area Manager was largely justified in passing you over. In which case, harsh as it may seem, the payoff for you is that you can blame someone else for your own shortcomings.

Another example might be Mrs Jones next door whom you dislike because she is often rude to her husband. Let us consider the payoff here. Perhaps Mr Jones is no angel and Mrs Jones is only giving as good as she gets. Be entirely honest. On reflection you realize that you've held a grudge against her ever since she asked you to move your car from across her driveway. The payoff here is that you can believe she made you move your car because she is a nasty woman, not because you knowingly parked it in the wrong place.

If you work through your resentments in this way, carefully and with absolute self-honesty, you will discover that a number of your resentments are unwarranted – in other words, there is another side to the story – and you can let them go. Others, while they may be entirely justified, give rise to emotions that you are not yet prepared to let go of. **Every resentment has a payoff, or else you wouldn't be hanging on to it.**

Frequently a resentment will be justified in that it is clear you have been mistreated in some way, sometimes grievously. Perhaps your Uncle Jack hit you when you were a child and you can see no way of letting go of your hurt and anger. Putting aside the rights or wrongs of his actions for a moment, ask yourself in all honesty how this resentment makes you feel. What is the payoff? Does it allow you to play victim? Does your anger about this give you a sense of power? Does it enable you to feel self-righteous? Does it leave you with a feeling of moral superiority?

Some people feel an instinctive resistance to this part of the clearing process, seemingly with good cause: 'So-and-so mistreated me and I'm supposed to be looking at **my** faults?' This is missing the point. Although we may get a dark pleasure from the payoff, the only ones who suffer when we 'refeel' resentments are ourselves, not the other people concerned.

The payoff is the mind's way of protecting itself, of creating positive emotions out of negative circumstances, but this process can be extremely clumsy and self-destructive. In the long run the payoff serves no purpose other than to create unhappiness.

Cost

In one of the examples given above your Area Manager passed you over for promotion and you feel angry. You have been able to establish that perhaps, on reflection, there might be another side to the story. Maybe the job went to a colleague because they were better qualified than you. It has become clear that you have cultivated the resentment not because it is justified but because it serves a useful purpose: it enables you to blame someone else for your lack of promotion.

In many instances you will find that your resentment will drop off at this point. You've looked at it with all the honesty and rationality you can muster and that does the trick, it's gone. You may actually feel the shift as it drops away. Some resentments, though, will still not budge that easily.

The general cost of resentments may be measured in terms of the effect that they have on our health, relationships and happiness. Pent-up negative emotions can give rise to all manner of physical ailments, from headaches and tiredness to backache. Every bit as damaging is the lowered sense of well-being and happiness that inevitably follows on from any resentment. Fears, anxieties and anger can give rise to varying degrees of irritability, depression and grumpiness. The people who suffer the most from these are ourselves and those who are closest to us.

There is a specific cost, too. In this case, the resentment towards your employer might also be affecting your job prospects. Where once you were upbeat and cheerful when it came to your dealings with your boss, since you were passed over for promotion you have become a little grumpy or un-responsive as if to say, 'I'll show you!' Rather than showing them how hard-working you can be, you are showing them your hurt and displeasure. Thus your Area Manager's per-ception of you – justified or not – as someone who didn't pull their weight as much as the person they promoted instead of you is now compounded by a belief that you are surly or aggressive. This further damages your prospects within the company and the downward cycle of the resentment continues. As a result you are passed over for promotion yet again and your resentment intensifies.

This may seem a fairly bleak picture but it is important not to underestimate the potentially destructive effects of pent-up negative emotions. Perhaps the cost of your resent-ment isn't as damaging or dramatic as the example given above but the pattern is often the same. Consider each resentment in turn and ask yourself what the cost is. Pride – 'I can't possibly change my attitude towards my boss after all this time, that would be a humiliating climb-down' – is not reason enough to hold on to a resentment. You are the person who will 'refeel' it and be damaged by it. Let it go . . . and it will release you.

False Assumptions

Every mind-clearing process has its surprises and its revela-tions. Let's go back to the scenario at the beginning of the chapter where your boyfriend dumped you, age 13. Imagine that you have worked on your resentment towards him and this, together with the passage of the years, means that you no longer feel anything much towards him. Certainly you no longer feel any anger. However, there is an association with his actions and a long-term fear of intimacy. In any situation like this, asking yourself some basic, common sense questions can break through the fear. For instance:

Why did he ditch me? He preferred another girl in my class.
Why did he prefer her? She was better, or prettier, than me.
Was she really? Well, of course, she must have been, or else
   he wouldn't have gone out with her.
How does this make you feel? Useless and inadequate. Ugly.
Anything else? I trusted him. He violated that trust.
How does that make you feel? Angry. Hurt. Useless.
Do you still feel that? Deep down, yes, I do.
*Is this feeling justified? Did Billy really drop you because you
   were ugly or useless, or was there another reason?* **Be
   entirely honest**. Well, he ditched that pretty girl in our
   class to go out with me, and after me he ditched the
   redhead for someone else. That's just the way it was.
   Come to think of it, at that age relationships rarely last
   more than a few months. So I don't suppose me being
   ugly or useless had anything to do with it.
*Is this self-image you have held on to for all these years – that
   you are a bit ugly and useless – in any way justified?* No.

Your perception at the time told you one thing and, because it has been held in your unconscious rather than your conscious mind, you have never questioned that belief – until now. Tell yourself the truth about the episode, out loud: 'He dropped me because he was a 13-year-old boy discovering girls for the first time and that is what 13-year-old boys (and girls) do. It had nothing whatever to do with me.' Let your false perception go. State it out loud: 'I was wrong, my mind misread the situation. I now know that I am **not** ugly or useless!'

Use the same process to work through each resentment in your inventory that still requires attention. Ask yourself:

What happened?
How does this make me feel?
Was/is my perception about this episode correct, or have
   I misread it?
What is the truth of the situation?
Am I now prepared to let go of my false perception?

Then make the conscious decision to let it go. It's that simple.

Svadyaya

Once you have completed your emotional detox, there is no need to repeat it. Any issues that come up can be dealt with on a daily basis during a period of daily self-study, or svadyaya. The word **svadyaya** translates as 'self-study'. It is an ancient practice from the Hindu tradition. At the end of each day allow yourself a few minutes to be alone and study your thoughts and actions over the past 24 hours or so. Svadyaya is a sort of emotional power shower and it is an invaluable tool for achieving long-term serenity and peace of mind.

During your daily svadyaya ask yourself the following questions:

Where have I been upset today and why?
Where others were at fault, what can I do to restore my
   peace of mind?
Where have I been selfish or unkind?
Where did I rush today and where was I at peace?
Have I taken proper care of myself both physically and
   spiritually?
Have I managed my time properly?
Have I been a responsible human being today?

A quicker way of completing svadyaya is to write down some headings on a card such as 'kindness', 'tolerance', 'resentments', 'patience', and so on. The emotional detox process will have drawn your attention to unskilful habits which you might want to add to this list, such as 'playing victim', perhaps, or 'dishonesty'. During svadyaya, simply run your eye down this list to see if any incidents spring to mind from the day and make a mental note of them.

Misunderstanding
If you pick up a resentment during the course of the day, begin by considering the possibility that you may have misread the situation. This need only take a moment. You might think: 'Joe completely ignored me when I met him by the coffee machine today. I don't think he likes me.' The truth of the matter is that Joe is exhausted at the moment and his mind was simply on other things. The majority of disagreements stem from misunderstandings. Considering

a resentment in this way is often enough to be able to let it go.

Understanding

If you can be sure that there was no misunderstanding in a given incident, try to see the other person's point of view. Perhaps Joe really did slight you by the coffee machine today. Ask yourself why he might have done so. Is there anything which might have triggered his behaviour? Perhaps he ignored you because you are quite often a little offhand with him, too? On the other hand, perhaps he is in awe of you – he might even fancy you or was feeling shy. As we have seen during the emotional detox, things aren't always how they outwardly appear. You will know you are making progress when your knee-jerk reaction to apparently selfish behaviour is to try to understand the other person's position rather than immediately responding with hurt or anger.

Effective communication

You have tried your hardest to understand why a person has behaved in a particular way and you are none the wiser. The next step is communication. Ask them in an entirely non-confrontational way about the episode: 'I hope I haven't upset you in some way, you seemed a little distracted when I saw you yesterday.' Whatever the answer you will be one step closer to resolving the issue. Properly handled, most difficult situations can be considerably improved by means of gentle, non-confrontational communication.

Emotional sickness

If you have considered all the options and it is clear that someone has, in fact, behaved badly towards you and that your resentment is to your mind justified, rather than being angry or resentful towards the other person try something new. Remember that bad behaviour is a soul-sickness in itself. We feel sorry for someone who is physically sick. Why not extend the same sympathy towards someone who is emotionally sick? If their behaviour is not reasonable or just then this is a person who is controlled by mean-spiritedness, fear or discouragement. Few things can be worse than to pass through life so afflicted.

One of the most effective ways of dispelling anger towards someone is to direct a loving prayer towards them. Sit quietly. Breathe and smile a half-smile. Contemplate the image of the person who has upset you and say something quietly to the image which is positive and uplifting, such as, 'I wish you health and happiness. May you one day master your fears.' Continue until you find compassion rising in your heart then gently bow your head towards the mental image you hold of them, in love and forgiveness. You may even picture a gentle embrace in which your feelings of com-passion are reciprocated. Repeat this process as often as you like until your negative emotions have dissipated. If you have never tried anything like this remember that often it is the thing which we least want to do that can have the most positive results.

Worries and Stressors

During the course of svadyaya you may become aware of certain anxieties that continue to come up. Now might be the time to address these. For example, your mind might return day after day to problems around a particular relationship or a financial difficulty. Anxieties such as these persist until we come up with solutions so jot the problems down in your notebook and think them through. Few people ever properly address their fears in this way; we tend to bury our heads in the sand and let our worries free-float over us. It may be that the problem is too big or complicated for you to resolve on your own, in which case you might want personal or professional advice from someone else. In this way you are taking control of the situation and during svadyaya you can work out what the best strategy might be for resolving the issue. This is also a good period of the day to consider what, if any, are the key stressors in your life. Noise? Environment? Lack of time? Decide what solutions you can implement to overcome these.

Not many people in contemporary Western society would even consider trying to get spiritually or emotionally fit. But achieving balance in your life means placing as much emphasis on your emotional equilibrium as on physical health. Emotional detoxing is absolutely crucial to this process.

When practised properly, svadyaya will help you let go of any negative emotions that may have arisen during the course of the day, thereby enabling you to keep your mind in a post-detox state of serenity and equilibrium. Like cleaning your teeth or painting your nails, your daily emotional cleansing need take only a couple of minutes. It is an excellent way to maintain a clear and easy consciousness, unclouded by anxiety and egoism. It is better to do a one-minute spot check at the end of the day while you brush your hair than an intensive half-hour workout which you tire of doing after a week. Allow yourself 'floating days' when you have a break from svadyaya, weekends and holidays, for example. You may choose to incorporate svadyaya as part of the Golden Hour which we have considered in chapter 1, 'Managing Your Life'. As we know, almost anyone can make time for that, if their priorities are in order!

Excessive contemplation can be counterproductive. The key here, as in all things, lies in equilibrium. Daily contemplation should be moderate rather than excessive, and counterbalanced with plenty of regular communication.

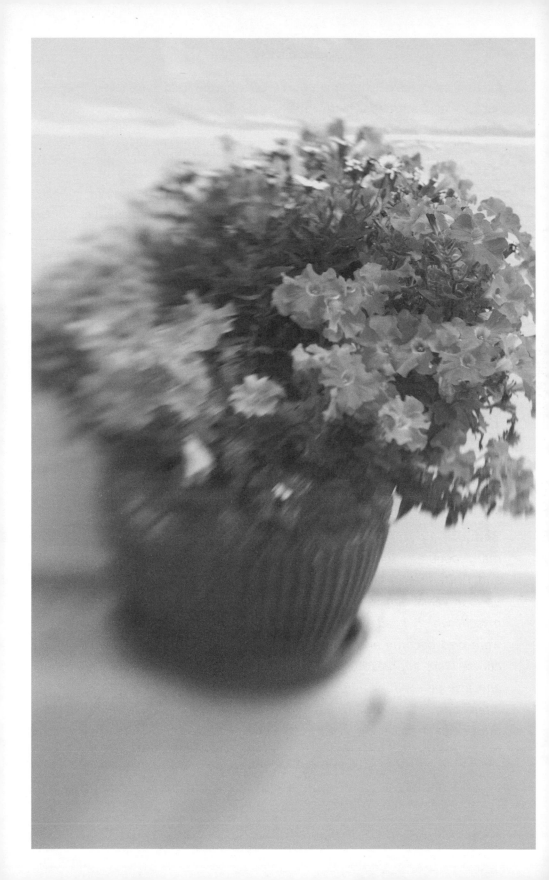

7 | Communication Skills

Heather: *Most of the disagreements in the world are due to misunderstandings, or failing to see the other person's point of view. Countless relationships – between nations and individuals – could be healed through proper communication. Communication skills are, without a doubt, amongst the most important skills that we can learn but very few of us are ever taught to communicate properly. While we spend years in the classroom learning algebra, geography and trigonometry, practically no time is devoted to the skilful tactics required for resolving disputes or effectively expressing our emotions.*

Ben: *The very idea of expressing our emotions is difficult for many people. I tend to have the opposite problem! Heather and I attended a corporate training day together about three or four years ago. I shared some fairly personal stuff about myself, which I felt was relevant at the time, but as the day wore on I became aware that most of the other people on the course were approaching the day from a far more professional, and less personal, standpoint! I felt a bit foolish and it was an interesting lesson in knowing where to draw the line between the personal and the professional. But Heather and I are good* *at communication – it comes fairly easily to both of us. I'm a trained counsellor and people tend to open up to me. Heather often gives her mobile number to people who are going through a difficult time.*

Heather: *I like to think that I am a good listener and I try to be there for friends and strangers alike – for example by visiting people who are going through the trauma of losing a limb. It's one thing to listen to someone else's problems and quite another skill to learn to share your own. I have to admit that I haven't always been the best communicator. I really had to work at it. I tended to hold back on what I wanted to say in case I hurt someone's feelings, which led to me becoming frustrated and expressing myself impatiently.*

Most people sit on their feelings. This can lead to negative emotions burrowing inwards, which can give rise to anxiety or neurosis, or else they are forced outwards and are often directed at the wrong person. Not only does effective communication reduce the risk of anger, neurosis or anxiety, it can also give us much needed objectivity. Sometimes it takes a third party to bring us to our senses.

If someone has upset you, run it past a friend. A sympathetic ear can work wonders in restoring your peace of mind and is an excellent way of letting off steam. Be careful, however, not to stack the facts in your favour. We've all done it, but if you give a friend an exaggerated and one-sided version of events it is quite possible that they will get angry on your behalf. This may sound great – it may be just what you wanted and you feel better in the short term – but it is more than likely to inflame the situation in the long term and then everyone suffers. Few things are as unreasonable or as destructive as a group of people making decisions based on a mixture of half-truths and lies. Groups, however small, are rarely as clear-thinking as individuals and as soon as people start taking sides you really lose any chance of a reasonable solution. When letting off steam, tread carefully and don't succumb to the temptation to exaggerate.

The key to effective communication is **how** it is done. Having shared your feelings with a friend, you may decide to discuss the matter with the person who has upset you. There is no harm in expressing hurt or anxiety in a manner which is calm, reasonable and does not point an accusatory finger. The advantage of talking directly to the other party is that it will give them an opportunity to rectify any misunderstandings that may have arisen, or to explain their point of view. If emotions are running high on either side or you feel that discussing it may make the situation even worse, it would be advisable only to express your feelings with someone else. You can always come back to the person you have fallen out with later if you choose to, when things have calmed down a little.

Mentors

We have already seen the importance of having someone to talk to while undertaking your emotional detox. Many people carry this through into their everyday lives. Divulging details about your personal life should, of course, be done with the right person and in the right circumstances. The same rules apply to finding someone to talk over everyday matters as applied to the person you chose to listen to your emotional detox. You might want to talk to a partner or spouse but it is generally better to have someone not quite so close to home who you can turn to in times of difficulty. Two-way exchanges are possible where people help each other but the best solution is often to find a 'mentor' who is kind and discreet, whose judgement you respect, and who in turn has someone else they can talk to when they need support.

You may prefer to share your feelings with a number of people. Friends and family will generally feel flattered if you go to them for help and feedback from time to time and they may welcome the opportunity it gives them to share their own issues with you in return.

Heather: *I am very fortunate. Not only do I have a very open and loving relationship with my husband, I also have a strong support network of twenty or so close girlfriends I know I can always turn to. Once a month or so we get together, kick off our shoes and sit in a circle talking about our lives and experiences. It's a wonderful opportunity to share negative feelings, help others to see the good in themselves and achieve a little balance. I don't know what I'd do without it. It is important with this sort of group sharing to be entirely honest. Sometimes my friends are good at recognizing when I am kidding myself or if I'm failing to see another person's point of view. None of us can be entirely objective when it comes to evaluating our own circumstances.*

Whether you go to a friend, your family or a mentor, the emotional support which sharing your feelings and anxieties can bring you will soon become a nurturing force in your life. You may decide to set up a support group, meeting perhaps weekly or monthly to share your experiences. There is nothing strange about group counselling, it is an entirely healthy process whereby we talk to other people as a means of releasing negative feelings and restoring a sense of perspective. If more of us drew on this valuable resource, fewer people would be dependent upon harmful emotional props such as comfort eating, drugs or cigarettes.

Honesty

When we are truly honest with another person we are being honest with ourselves. Self-honesty lies at the heart of self-acceptance and without it lasting happiness is impossible. We all have good and bad points. Being open about these with someone else can be a very powerful tool in self-acceptance. Ask yourself: 'What sort of person would I be if there were no praise and no blame?' Try to be that person with your mentor. If you can let just one person in, the rest will follow. The most terrifying thing is to accept yourself completely. If you can truly be yourself with another person you are half way there.

Listening

Communication is as much about listening to others as it is about expressing your own feelings. It is all very well drawing on the love and support of others but we must be prepared to do the same when people need us. As with most things, it is all a question of balance: don't hesitate to turn to others if you need their help and support but if people around you are unhappy or in trouble, try to be there for them, too.

If someone turns to you for support the best that you can do is to share your own experience, where appropriate, and try to act as a sounding board to assist them in reaching their own conclusions. Be wary of imparting advice, however. Mostly all anyone wants is to let off a little steam in a sympathetic ear. Allow them to make their own decisions wherever possible.

There is often a temptation to tell people what they want to hear to make them feel better, regardless of the facts. If you do this, be very careful not to inflame a situation and always bear in mind that what you are hearing is probably only half the story. This is particularly true where someone wants your advice over a personal disagreement of some sort. Be sympathetic, of course, but even if your instincts are crying out for you to protect your friend and you can feel yourself getting angry on their behalf, try not to. It will only intensify their anger. Guide them instead towards standing up for themselves in a calm and rational manner (nobody says we should all become doormats) and then help them to let go of their emotions.

One of the most effective ways of doing this is by following the skills outlined in the emotional detox chapter. Someone turns to you for advice. They outline their problem and you offer them a sympathetic ear. Occasionally your input will need to be more significant. You might want to explore with them the possibility that a misunderstanding may have given rise to their hurt, fear or anger. If it is clear that this is not the case, help them to understand the other person's behaviour by looking at the opposite perspective. Finally, help them to evaluate whether action needs to be taken to improve the situation or whether they might be better off acknowledging the lack of emotional skill of the other party and simply walking away. Sometimes walking away is the most intelligent response.

Protecting Yourself

When listening to someone, try not to absorb their energy. If they are speaking angrily and quickly, are you responding by also talking fast? The fascinating thing with both verbal and non-verbal communication is how they rub off on to other people. If you smile at someone they will generally smile back. Likewise if you scowl. On an unconscious level we tend to mirror image the body language of people around us: we fold our arms, cross our legs or yawn in response to other people's own arm folding, leg crossing or yawning! There is something deeply rooted in the human mind which leads us to do this. On the one hand this means that we have some influence over the face the world shows us because, by and large, it's the same face that we show to the world. On the other hand, if you are trying to remain neutral when the person talking to you is highly emotional, you need to be aware of whether you are copying their mannerisms and getting sucked into the drama of the situation. Keep a close eye on your breathing. Inhale slowly and calmly as this will help you to remain detached.

Using communication skills effectively as a resource to release negative energies is one of the most important things that anyone can learn. By the same token you should also learn when to cut people loose. If someone doesn't make the effort to fight back a little, if they become over-dependent upon you, you are not doing them or yourself any favours.

Give them your time and your support but don't allow them to rely completely on you.

Your Amends List

During the emotional detox you drew up an inventory of people who have hurt you and you worked through that list. You also listed the people that you might have done harm to. This is an area which we have not yet examined – the people to whom you feel you might owe amends.

Look back over the whole of your emotional detox inventory and underline the names of all the people you feel you may have been unkind or unfair to in some way. Expand your inventory by going back in your mind as far as you can and adding the names of anyone else you can think of whom you may have significantly mistreated.

The likelihood is that most of these incidents are so inconsequential or happened so long ago that they now seem irrelevant. What needs to be acknowledged is the draining effect that accumulated guilt can have on your energy levels and sense of well-being.

Making Amends

It may be that there is a long-running feud between yourself and a friend or a relative which neither of you has handled particularly skilfully. The last thing you may feel like doing is apologizing for your part in years of fallout. But making amends isn't necessarily about apologizing.

Aunt Sally is an interfering and unpleasant woman and you tend to bad-mouth her whenever she comes up in the conversation. You can combat negative thoughts about someone by making positive statements about them. You can begin your 'amends' to her by seeing her as someone who is emotionally unwell rather than plain vindictive. Consider the validity of this assertion in Aunt Sally's case and set aside a few minutes to send her a healing prayer as described in the emotional detox chapter. Then resolve not to speak ill of her again, any more than you would speak ill of someone because of a physical ailment they have. Try to mend the relationship with her in your heart so that the anger and hurt you carry around from it (however small it may be) entirely disappears.

In the course of a lifetime most of us will have done things we regret. Maybe you were less than honest in your dealings with another person and they have suffered as a consequence, or perhaps you neglected someone at a time when they needed you. It's never too late to make your peace. A well-crafted letter or a carefully planned phone call can sweep away years of ill-feeling and contacting people you have lost touch with is becoming increasingly easy through the internet.

In the majority of cases you will be surprised at the welcome response you receive. It may well be that the person you approach has no recollection of any harm done, in which case they will be very surprised to receive an apology. Or, if they do remember, they will probably be delighted that you have approached them in this way.

On other occasions you may find that your advances are rejected. Perhaps you have apologized to your neighbour for your part in a long-running dispute. Rather than acknowledging their part in events they may instead take this as an admission that you were wrong and they were right. As long as you are not apologizing for standing up for your rights but only for those things said or done which you genuinely believe were wrong of you, then you have done your bit. Don't try to control their response to your approach and on no account point the accusatory finger. Remember that we are responsible only for our own attitudes and behaviour. Simply make your amends and leave it at that. It does not mean that you are going to stop standing up for your rights just because you have demonstrated a degree of humility.

Here lies the key to this exercise. The whole purpose of making amends to someone else is to make **you** feel better. The fact that the other person may benefit as well is a side-issue. But regardless of how they respond, be careful not to launch into an offensive about their part in what happened. This is about clearing your side of the street, not theirs. Try not to get drawn into any conversations about who was right or wrong. It is generally enough to tell them you simply wish to apologize for your part in the disagreement and leave it at that.

It may be that you have done things which would be harmful to other people if you were to disclose them. If you have had an affair that has long been over, would your partner be hurt if you told them? You have no right to risk other people's happiness or sense of security in order to make yourself feel better. An appropriate amends in such a case may simply be a decision not to behave in this way again.

The Payback

The whole process of making amends is difficult to understand unless you have undertaken it. At first sight it looks both unappealing and unnecessary. Why bother apologizing for things that are in the past and over which you have no control? This is essentially an experiential process, once you have experienced it you will realize its significance. Give it a try, once, and see how you feel. The process can be extremely powerful. Most people who have applied themselves to the process walk away feeling much lighter.

Having made your amends, you can keep the emotional pipework clean by being mindful of your behaviour in future. If your inventory suggests that you have a tendency to behave in a certain way, continue to make amends to those around you by breaking these behaviour habits. Ultimately, it is you who benefits from this – by becoming a happier, kinder and more open person.

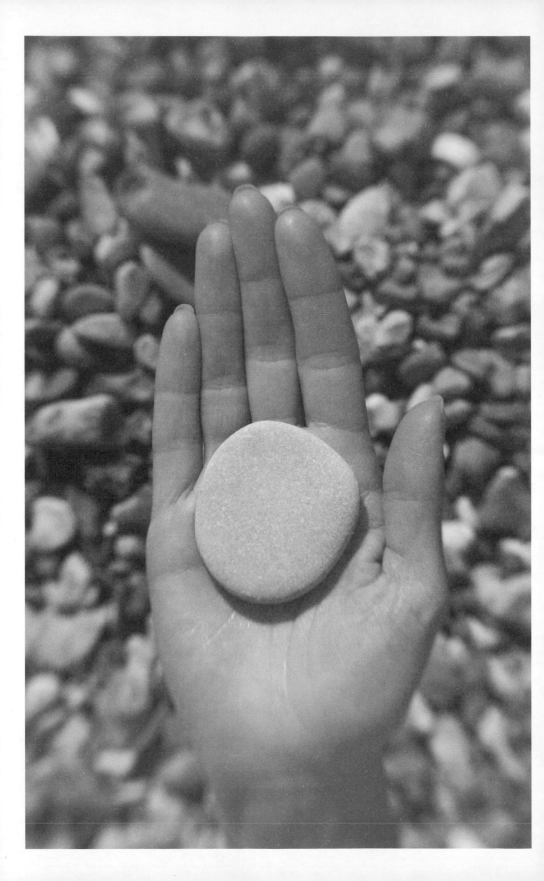

8 | Meditation

Heather: *I never appreciated the value of slowing down and taking life as it comes when I was in my teens or twenties. After I lost my leg I tried meditation as a means of relaxing but it wasn't much use. I couldn't sit still for more than a couple of minutes, my mind was in overdrive worrying about all the things I had to get on with. Yet I stuck with it. Nowadays I manage my time more effectively so I don't feel the same sense of stress and urgency and I suppose I am a calmer person – possibly due in part to regular meditation. Sitting still comes much more easily to me. I meditate on a deck in the garden in the summer and in winter I sit on a yoga mat on the sitting-room floor. If I don't have time to meditate in the morning then I make time at the end of the day, generally last thing before going to bed. So I don't want to hear you say: 'But I don't have time!'*

Ben: *There is no doubt that meditation can transform and enrich your life. The Tibetan teacher Sogyal Rinpoche said: 'The gift of learning to meditate is the greatest gift you can give your-self.' One of the hardest things for me to understand was that I could not expect immediate results from just a few meditation sessions. I have found, however, that by continuing a daily* *practice the payback has been deep and lasting. Nowadays I feel more calm and I am better able to deal with stress. I am quite sure that this is because of regular meditation. The main benefit for me has been a deep sense of inner 'connection' – to whom or what I don't know exactly. Once meditation became a regular habit I began to really look forward to those few minutes at the beginning of each day in which I could make this connection.*

Meditation has been practised in the East for over 3000 years and it is perhaps the most ancient spiritual practice of humankind. It has become increasingly popular in the West since the Maharaja Mahesh Yogi brought it to public attention in the 1960s and it now has several million adherents in both Europe and North America. The only mystery is how it took so long to become so popular.

Brainwave monitoring suggests that during meditation the brain produces evenly balanced alpha and theta brainwave rhythms, an ideal state where the body is relaxed and the mind calm but alert. In other studies, people who meditate regularly have reported an improvement in their relationships, marital satisfaction and academic performance – it has even been said to boost IQ. One scientific study followed over 2000 meditators for a period of five years. Amongst other things it found that meditators over the age of 40 spent 70% less time in hospital and made 74% fewer visits to their doctors than non-meditators. An increasing number of GPs are encouraging patients with stress-related ailments to take up meditation as a complement to conventional treatment. A recent study reported in *Which?* magazine concluded that meditators were biologically several years younger than non-meditators. Whilst it might reasonably be argued that the sort of people who meditate regularly probably look after themselves in other ways too, it is difficult to think of a single product on the open market which can lay claim to such impressive results.

East and West

The positive effects of meditating are very powerful but it takes a while to master. In the Eastern tradition, meditation is seen as a means of reaching 'enlightenment', a state of absolute bliss which is said to come about when the mind of the individual is merged with that of the collective unconscious. This is a process known as **samadhi**, which translates literally as 'to merge'. At its most basic, meditation can give you a deeply rooted sense of warmth, security and an inner calmness which remains with you as you go about your everyday life.

The spiritual aspect of meditation puts some people off, but there is no reason whatsoever to feel wary. You're not going anywhere when you meditate, except inward for greater peace of mind. You are always in control. Meditation is about being awake; you are not asleep, in a trance state, or communicating with spirits. And, contrary to what some people say, meditation is not in conflict with Christian teaching. Christianity, Judaism and Islam have all taught meditative practices. You can practise any religion or no religion at all and still derive the full benefits of meditation.

If you're still not convinced that meditation is for you, try it out for three or four weeks and see what difference, if any, it makes to your life.

Getting Started

Meditation is a very simple process. You don't need any specialist equipment or training and it can be done almost anywhere. You might find it helpful to create a special or 'sacred' space in a corner of your sitting room or bedroom with candles, incense or fresh flowers. The smell of incense can be effective for creating the right atmosphere but make sure you choose one you like as some incense sticks can be fairly pungent.

Try to find a regular time for your meditation, a slot when you know you can keep a few minutes clear. First thing in the morning is good, before breakfast, as it sets you up for the rest of the day. Meditating after a heavy meal can be difficult as you may find yourself nodding off. You will also find it difficult to apply yourself properly when things are frantic or when you are over-stimulated by caffeine or alcohol.

Meditation tends to exaggerate your mood. If you're depressed or anxious, meditation may concentrate these feelings and make them worse so try to choose a time of day when you are feeling positive or upbeat. If you are not a morning person it may be sensible to meditate later in the day. A good rule of thumb is: 'If you're down, move around. Feeling great? Meditate!'

Short, regular sessions are more effective than long, infrequent sittings. Begin with brief meditation segments – five minutes maximum – for the first two weeks. You can then increase the length of each session to ten minutes for the next fortnight, and to fifteen or twenty minutes a day thereafter.

You may prefer to meditate in silence but not everyone

responds well to this and some people like to play music or natural sound cassettes such as dolphins, waves or rain. Unless you live in a bunker there will be noises and outside interruptions while you meditate but with practice you'll be able to ignore them. You should, however, turn off the phone and your mobile and let the people you live with know in advance when you are not to be disturbed.

Wear comfortable clothing (baggy trousers and a sweat-shirt, for example) and remove your shoes. If you're too hot or cold during your session you will find it impossible to switch off so adjust the heating, open or close windows, and so on. Strong light, too, can be a distraction so dim over-head lights or turn them off. Spend a few minutes before each session creating the right environment. Once you have settled down to meditate the last thing you will want to do is keep getting up to remove ticking clocks or to close windows.

Finding Your Best Position

The drawback to meditating flat on your back is that you might fall asleep. You may prefer sitting on a hard chair with your back supported, feet together and your hands resting lightly on your lap. Or sit cross-legged on the floor, resting your hands on your lap or on your knees, keeping your body upright and your arms relaxed. However you sit, imagine that the top of your head is suspended from the ceiling by a piano wire and you will automatically assume an upright posture.

The cross-legged position is traditionally seen as the standard or 'correct' posture for meditation, but what matters is that you find a posture which suits you. Play around with various positions and settle on the one that feels most comfortable. It is not necessary to 'work up' to the cross-legged position.

Breathing Meditation

Settle yourself into your comfortable position, close your eyes and focus your attention on your breathing. Don't expect anything extraordinary to happen. Just enjoy the stillness. Every few seconds your attention will be distracted by thoughts or sounds. When these distractions arise, gently let them go then turn your attention once more to your breathing.

Be aware of the rhythm of your breath. Try to focus on this. Don't alter your breathing pattern, simply watch the ebb and flow of your breath as it flows in and out of your body. Then start counting your breaths – inhale, exhale, 'one', inhale, exhale, 'two', and so on. Count up to ten, allowing yourself to become a little mesmerized, then begin another cycle. Every time you find your mind drifting off in another direction, focus on your breathing and start again at 'one'. For the first few weeks you will find it difficult to get beyond three or four before your mind begins to wander. That's okay. Be patient and just keep on counting.

Many people make an effort to be peaceful. Don't make any effort to be anything. Just breathe as you find it and be as you are. Your breathing will become shallower and slower as you become more relaxed. Put aside every plan, every project, and be in the moment. The world will still be there when you finish your meditation. There is nothing wrong with setting an alarm to bring you back to reality if you are worried about your session overrunning. Don't be overly solemn or feel that you are taking part in some special ritual. Let go of the idea that you are meditating. Just breathe.

Session Segments

In the beginning, break your meditation session into small, manageable chunks. Sit in your comfortable position, close your eyes and take a few really deep breaths. With each breath draw as much air into your belly as you can and try to make each outgoing breath last a few seconds longer than the incoming breath. If you focus your attention on the outgoing breath you will find that your incoming breath will automatically become deeper. If your mind is crowded with thoughts, that's fine. Allow them to come, and don't try to dispel them. You haven't started meditating yet, this is just your warm-up and it is a good opportunity for stray thoughts to express themselves. By the time you start meditating, in a few moments, many of the thoughts that bubbled up to the surface will already have come and gone.

Open your eyes. Now is your opportunity to get rid of an itch or stretch tense muscles. In the early stages of meditating you will feel the urge to scratch or move every few seconds. Within a few weeks the 'itch urge' will begin to disappear.

Close your eyes. Begin your breathing exercise. Stay with it for a few minutes then open your eyes. Fidget or stretch your limbs if needs be. Now close your eyes again. Focus on the moment. Don't waste time with mental wanderings, simply enter the silence within. Stay in this space for five minutes or so, then open your eyes.

You might like to end each meditation session with a couple of minutes' relaxation, lying flat on your back in what is called the 'Corpse Position'. Allow the weight of your body to increase and be aware of the floor beneath you supporting you. Then slowly open your eyes and presto! You're ready to face the day.

Mantras and Candle Meditations

A mantra is a word or phrase which is repeated aloud. It is another way of focusing on your breath. Perhaps the most popular word used in meditation across the globe is the Sanskrit **Om**. Chanting 'Om' is said to put you in tune with the universe as it is believed to be the basis of all sounds. However, a mantra can be any word, sound or phrase, in any language and people often make up their own mantras.

If you decide to use a mantra, breathe deeply and exhale slowly and evenly. Chant your mantra as loudly as you dare so that you can feel its vibration resonating in your chest. Then gradually lower the volume, looping the word or phrase into a cycle of sound so that the end of the mantra blends in with the beginning. Imagine yourself going deeper and deeper within yourself as you chant. With even intonation and rhythm the process becomes fairly mesmerizing. You're bound to feel a little stupid or awkward at first but if you can get over that it is definitely worth trying.

A popular alternative to counting your breath or chanting a mantra is candle or flame meditation. Sit two or three feet away from a lighted candle with the flame at or slightly below eye level. If you feel cross-eyed move a little further back. Blink a few times in rapid succession and fix your eyes on the flame.

114

Meditation

Look at the flame for as long as you can without blinking. When your eyes begin to water and you need to blink, do so then resume your gaze. Acknowledge every thought that comes into your mind and then let it go.

This ancient practice (known as **trataka**) strengthens inner vision. Over the centuries it has been practised by spiritual sages and monks across all the continents. It is considered to be one of the most powerful forms of meditation.

To the uninitiated meditation sounds fairly easy yet it can be surprisingly difficult because your mind is constantly distracted by a steady stream of thoughts. Mastering this gets easier with time and regular practice. It can take several weeks before you begin to feel the benefits of meditation and perhaps because of this the greatest obstacle facing many people who take up meditation is, quite simply, boredom.

Visualization

One of the most effective ways of getting into the habit of regular meditation without even a hint of boredom is visualization. At its most basic this can mean closing your eyes and transporting yourself to a positive or nurturing environment – a sun-drenched beach, for example, or in front of a roaring fire in a cosy log cabin deep inside a forest. Visualization can be both engrossing and enjoyable, and as such it can be a highly effective way of getting into the habit of sitting down in silence for a few minutes each day. When you find that you are really enjoying this brief break from the hurly-burly of life you can gradually replace visualization with 'no thought' exercises such as focusing on the breath, mantra or candle flame meditation.

Here are some visualization exercises that you might find helpful. With each one, read it through two or three times before you begin and then recreate the exercise in your own way.

Visualization Exercise 1

We will begin with a fairly straightforward exercise. Sit comfortably and close your eyes. Take a few really deep breaths. Imagine you are sitting on a beach. The sand beneath you is warm and you can hear waves breaking on the shore. The sun is bathing everything in warmth and light and there is a gentle breeze. 'Lose' yourself in this scene – picture the sights, sounds and smells of the beach. After a few minutes open your eyes and return to the present.

You can choose any location or environment that you wish: a mountaintop overlooking a lush green valley, or even a scene from your childhood such as your parents' sitting room on the night before Christmas. Take a couple of minutes to lose yourself in the scene. Use all of your senses. What can you smell? Mulled wine, perhaps, or the Christmas tree? What can you hear? Christmas carols playing on the radio in the kitchen? Try to visualize as many aspects of the scene as you can. Perhaps a long-gone but much-loved family pet is curled up on the carpet beside you. For a few moments really allow yourself to **be** there.

The scene can be as idealized as you wish – a family gathering free from any family arguments, or a beach without sunburn and the roar of nearby traffic. Above all, the location must be one which is attractive to you and one in which you can completely lose yourself for a few minutes. With

116

practice this will get easier. You can undertake this form of visualization almost anywhere.

Visualization Exercise 2

This visualization exercise can be used if you are suffering physical pain and is particularly effective for headaches.

Sit comfortably. Close your eyes. Take a few really deep breaths. Focus on the location of your pain. Picture its size and shape – for example, if you have a headache at the front left-hand side of your forehead, visualize its length and width. Now give it colour. Is it a throbbing purple, perhaps, or dark red, or a softer mustard colour?

Once you have pictured in your mind the colour, size and shape of your pain, breathe in deeply and imagine that you are breathing in a pure, white, mist-like breath of positive energy. Picture this healing air going to the very centre of the pain and swirling around like a vapour. Picture the white vapour changing colour as it mixes with the pain. With each out breath, allow the pain to be discharged with your breath through your mouth. In your mind's eye see coloured vapour flow from your lips. Continue this process until the pain has dissipated.

Visualization is a highly effective tool for overcoming stress and creating a sense of inner security and well-being. As you practise this more and more you will be able to enter into the silence within yourself without difficulty. When this begins to happen you should notice a gradual change in your outlook and your responses to everyday situations. You will catch yourself facing stressful situations with a calmness and a clarity of mind which at first seems out of character.

Lose Yourself

You don't only have to 'visualize' with your mind, you can use your other senses, too. Close your eyes and smell a flower. What impression does this have on you? Smell it again and really lose yourself in the aroma of the flower. Or place four or five treats on a plate: an olive, for example, or a slice of mango or a sweet. Put each piece of food in your mouth by turn. Really experience its flavour, aroma and texture as if for the first time. Make the experience of each last as long as you can. When you can no longer resist the temptation to bite, fully enjoy the flavour-burst. Try to lose yourself in the experience entirely.

Go outside on a clear, mild day. Spread a coat or blanket on the grass, lie on your back and gaze at the sky. What do you see? Animals? Witches? People? Allow your imagination to take over for a few minutes and lose yourself in the sky.

Mini-Meditations

Many people simply don't have the time to fit a meditation session into their daily schedule. Of course, it might be argued that the busier and more stressed you are the more you need to meditate! If clearing a window of a few minutes really is out of the question you can do little mini-meditations during the day, when you are sitting in the dentist's waiting room, for example, or being held in a phone queue. Close your eyes, sit upright, and plant both feet firmly on the floor. Then breathe. The magic lies in the very last drop of breath – the top-up – so fill your lungs until they are completely full and allow your muscles to relax with each successive out breath. This should have an immediate and fairly profound effect on your sense of well-being.

In the Zen tradition there is a saying: 'If you want a small enlightenment, go to the country. If you want a big enlightenment, go to the city.' The skilful meditator takes the world as he finds it and the more challenging the environment the more it has to teach you. If you can learn to meditate to the sounds of a train your daily commute can become one of the most relaxing parts of your day. Of course, travelling by train can be both exhausting and demanding and there will be days when it will be as much as you can do to find a place to stand let alone switch off and find a peaceful inner oasis. But there will also be journeys where you find yourself wishing you had a few more stops to go.

Meditation may be one of the greatest gifts you can give yourself but it doesn't magically deliver results. The key to successful meditation is – in the words of the famous violinist who was asked by a stranger how you get to Carnegie Hall – practise, practise, practise. Break your practice in gradually and give yourself time to get into the habit. The results are worth waiting for. Don't stop before the miracle happens.

More than material success, more even than physical health, emotional well-being is for many people the keystone of happiness. No matter how carefully you manage your life, how 'successful' you are in material terms, or how single-minded you are in achieving a healthy lifestyle, if you don't take care of your mind you may never reach your full potential for happiness.

The third essential key to a lifetime of well-being:

BODY BALANCE

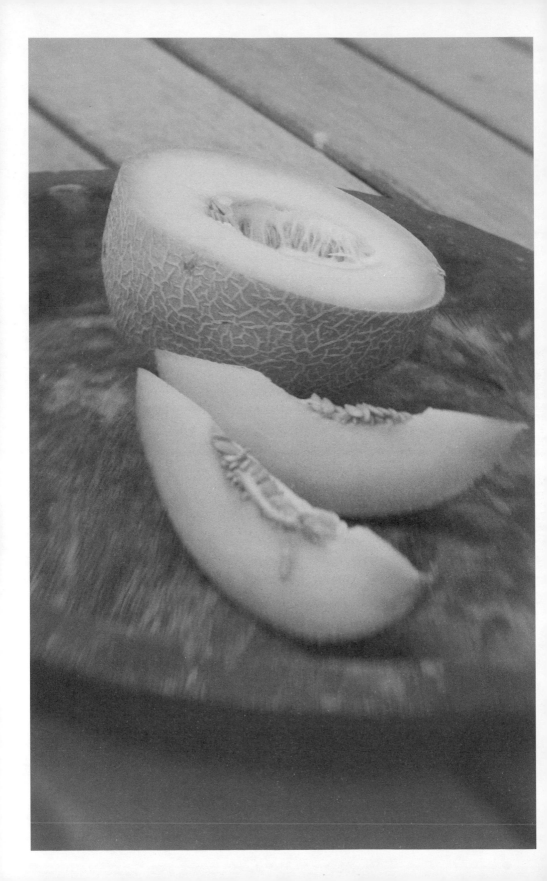

9 | Nutrition

Heather: *When I was younger and modelling, I was always being told that I was five or six pounds overweight. I tried every diet – the Hay Diet, the Grapefruit Diet, you name it. By the time I was 27 I had decided that diets are not for me: They would work for a while, I would lose a few pounds, but I would always end up putting it all back on again. I call these my yo-yo years! Nowadays, eating for me is about eating for health not for staying thin. By eating a sensible, healthy diet and taking regular exercise I keep my weight stable. I've been the same weight for ten years now – ever since I gave up dieting! If I lose too much weight my leg digs into the artificial limb, which can be extremely uncomfortable. Conversely, if I put on too much weight my leg begins to swell and I start getting phantom pains. I don't really believe in diets but I am a firm believer in healthy eating and plenty of exercise to keep my weight at the right level.*

When I was in hospital the food was terrible and I couldn't get rid of an infection. A girlfriend told me that she had recovered from a serious illness at a place called the Hippocrates Health Institute in America. I checked myself in and one of the first things they did was teach me the health benefits of a vegetarian diet. Initially, therefore, I took up a vegetarian diet purely because of my health. My concern for the welfare of animals came some time later.

These days I really take care of what I put into my body and have become a vegan. I planned it for six months and went on to the viva.org.uk website. They have a shop from which I ordered my Belgian chocolate, vegan chicken, garlic sausage slices, and stilton and cranberry cheese. Planning in advance – not just becoming a vegan overnight – made it much easier. I love things like couscous, salads, roast vegetables, pasta and risotto. One of the staples of my diet is oatmeal which sustains blood sugar levels for many hours. At times in my monthly cycle I indulge myself a little by eating chocolate. Much Belgian chocolate is vegan as it contains 70% cocoa and no milk. I reckon that as I'm self-disciplined for most of the rest of the month it's important that I'm not too hard on myself. A little of what you enjoy most can do you a power of good. I used to eat so much chocolate that friends told me I was a chocoholic and perhaps they were right – it wasn't unusual for me to consume six or seven bars of chocolate in a day. I paid for it, of course, not only in terms of my weight and the condition of my skin but in low energy levels and poor self-esteem. I now understand that the food you eat is the cornerstone of a healthy lifestyle.

Ben: *That's probably true, but it's not easy, is it? I remember Heather once pulling me up for eating a Mars bar for breakfast. I have found changing my diet extremely difficult. I don't drink or smoke, and food is a real pleasure for me. I can spend a week or so eating well but then I will walk past a deli and all my good intentions go to pot. I became a vegetarian two or three years* *ago but I've always loved the taste of meat and it all got too much for me when I found myself walking past the spit-roasted chickens in our local supermarket. I bought one and devoured it in a single sitting. It was factory farmed, it was greasy, but boy, was it delicious! Heather suggested I drink a protein shake each morning and took me to a health food shop to show me the vegetarian meat alternatives – sausages, bacon, 'pork' joints, all sorts of food. I found that it is almost impossible to differentiate between many of these and meat. As a result I have pretty much succeeded in sticking to my diet ever since.*

Imagine buying an expensive new limousine – a car designed to be run on high-grade unleaded petrol – and filling the tank with low-grade tractor fuel. This is what many people do to their bodies. Instead of eating wholesome, natural, delicious food we pack ourselves full of pesticides, toxins and junk. Eating a poor diet is so endemic in our society that few people realize they could significantly increase their performance and energy levels simply by changing what they eat.

Macro and Micronutrients

The energy value of food is measured in calories. A moderately active man of between 19 and 50 years requires a daily intake of 2550 calories; a woman requires 1940 calories. Having said that, unless you are genetically predisposed to being overweight or you suffer from a thyroid problem or similar difficulties, it is fair to say that if you eat sensibly and take regular exercise you can completely forget about counting calories.

The human body takes in calories in the form of carbo-hydrates, fat and protein (and alcohol). These are what are known as the three **macronutrients** ('big foods'). Macro-nutrients provide us with energy and, in the case of protein, they provide the body with the structural elements of growth and tissue repair. The body also needs tiny quantities of **micronutrients** ('little foods') such as vitamins, minerals and protective phytochemicals which bolster the body's defence system.

Don't get too bogged down in exactly how much of which macro or micronutrients your diet should consist of. There is, in fact, considerable debate amongst doctors and nutrition-ists as to what constitutes a 'healthy' diet. Instead, let's focus on what foodstuffs are generally agreed to be good to eat, and which ones you would be wise to avoid.

Things to Enjoy

Vegetables

Ideally, around 40% of the food you eat should be in the form of vegetables. Over-cooking vegetables depletes them of their vitamin and mineral content so lightly cook them or, best of all, eat lots of them raw. Raw vegetable juices are great for detoxifying your system.

Whole grains

Grains such as wheat, barley, rye, oats and rice provide us with many of the basic elements of human nutrition. Try to eat short grain, organically grown brown rice fairly regularly. The body slowly breaks rice down into glucose which is steadily released into the bloodstream to give you sustained energy. Any unused glucose is stored in the liver and naturally released later in the day if your energy levels fall. It is therefore an ideal food for keeping blood sugar levels – and energy levels – stable. If you're new to brown rice, cook it for a little longer than you would cook white rice. Gradually, as you get used to it, reduce the cooking time. Cooked rice will keep for about two days if stored in the fridge. It can also be frozen.

Fruit

Most people eat far too little fruit. We should all be having seven to ten portions of fresh fruit and veg a day as they are packed with antioxidants that fight diseases – from heart disease to prostate cancer.

Water

Taking in plenty of water is the best way to rid your body of the toxins it picks up throughout the day. The kidneys, liver and digestive tract all benefit. Drink your fill of bottled or filtered water but do remember that most foods contain a quantity of water, especially raw vegetables, so don't feel compelled to drink litres and litres of water daily if this doesn't feel right for you. One litre a day when you are eating plenty of fruits and vegetables is probably enough. Try to sip water continuously throughout the day. You'll be surprised how many litres this adds up to.

Heather: *Guzzling a litre in one go, like my friend Suzie after her weekly hangover, only means we have to stop the car three times on our journey to the country.*

There is a popular misconception that purified or distilled water has been robbed of its mineral content. This is an unfortunate belief as the benefits of purifying water are significant. Unfiltered tap water contains a host of toxins and pollutants which are best avoided.

Protein and the vegetarian diet

Heather: *Many people are shocked when I tell them there is more protein in 100 calories of broccoli than in 100 calories of steak.*

The biggest obstacle people have to giving up meat is that they think their diet will lack protein. Your protein needs are automatically met by a balanced, varied vegetarian diet (there is even protein in potatoes). Adherents to the Atkins Diet will be relieved to learn that it is entirely possible to have a high-protein, low-carb diet without eating any meat. Protein-rich foods include nuts and seeds; veggie burgers and sausages; and soya products such as tofu. Plus pulses such as baked beans, chick peas, lentils, kidney beans and, you may be surprised to learn, cereal, rice, pasta and whole-meal bread. Baked beans on toast is an excellent meal. Take heed if you're on a low-carb track. The World Health Organization says that 50–70% of our diet should contain complex carbohydrates (brown rice, whole wheat pasta, oats, etc.) if we want to remain healthy.

Omega-3s

In the 1970s, scientists made an association between omega-3 fatty acids and human health while studying the Inuit people of Greenland. It was observed that the Inuit suffered far less from diseases such as coronary heart disease and rheumatoid arthritis than most other cultures, despite the fact that their diet is very high in whale, salmon and seal fat. It was observed that these foods are all rich in omega-3 fatty acids – a form of polyunsaturated fat.

Omega-3s are found in the membrane of every cell in the body and they are used in the regulation of all biological functions including those of the cardiovascular, nervous and immune systems. We need them for the optimal functioning of just about every bodily process. It has been proven that a good intake of Omega-3s is a natural anti-depressant.

Omega-3s can be obtained in capsule form from most high street chemists. Vegetarian Omega-3 capsules are also freely available and foods such as flaxseed oil, walnuts and green, leafy veg are good sources.

Things to Avoid

People who eat well have fantastic levels of energy. However, if you adopt an optimum diet and you still feel lethargic it may be that you suffer from a food intolerance. Certain foods common to our diet are energy sappers and many people suffer from intolerances to them without being aware of it.

The easiest way to establish if you suffer from an allergy or intolerance is to consult an allergy specialist. If you suspect an intolerance, first thing in the morning take your pulse or temperature before eating a food you believe you may have a problem with. If your temperature or pulse increases after eating the food this can be a sign of an intolerance. Don't worry too much, many allergies or intolerances are temporary but it is a good idea to discuss your findings with your doctor.

Wheat

Wheat is generally seen to be wholesome and healthy but for a great many people its advantages are outweighed by its disadvantages. Wheat contains a substance called gluten to which many people are intolerant to one degree or another. Gluten intolerance can cause constipation, diarrhoea or wind. Excessive gluten intake is also a common cause of tiredness, depression and irritability. Bread, biscuits, pasta, cereals, cakes and flour all contain wheat. Other grains which contain gluten are barley, rye and oats, although oats are generally much more easily tolerated than wheat. Eat foods containing wheat sparingly, perhaps once a day.

Dairy produce

Cow's milk has the reputation of being an essential source of calcium. However, you will get all the calcium your body needs if you eat enough fresh fruit, vegetables and pulses. Professor T. Colin Campbell shows in *The China Study* how the consumption of cow's milk can lead to Type 1 diabetes early in life and many cancers and other diseases later on in life. Cow's milk is for baby cows, and even they won't touch it after they are a year old.

Heather: *One of the most shocking facts I discovered, and it is proven scientifically, is that there is pus in cow's milk – and it's legal – up to 400 million pus cells per litre of milk in the UK, and 500 million as a legal maximum in the US. Imagine chomping on pus in your latte.*

There are many cow's milk alternatives, such as rice milk, hazelnut milk, almond milk, oat milk, soya milk and pea milk, readily available in health food stores and supermarkets. Just make sure they are pure, with no added sugars or fats. It's simple to make your own – for nut milk simply combine one part nuts to three parts water, blend well and strain – and you can use the leftover pulp to make a great cake. It's so quick and means you have fresh milk every morning. Test them all until you find one you love, and next time you go to Starbucks be sure to get a Soya Latte!

Butter is very high in saturated fat, the kind that is implicated in raised cholesterol levels. There are many healthy olive oil or vegetable oil alternatives. Cheese is also a major source of these undesirable fats, even low-fat cheese, so eat it sparingly. If you wish to avoid milk but love the taste of yoghurt or cheese, try the new soya-based brands.

Meat

If you choose to eat meat, avoid all factory-farmed produce. Apart from the ethical considerations the chemicals which are pumped into factory-farmed meat and fish are horrific. All meat, even 'organic', 'free-range' meats, contain sizeable amounts of cholesterol, saturated fats and animal protein – which is harder on the kidneys than plant protein. Meat also lacks fibre, vitamins beta carotene, C and E (the antioxidants that protect us from Western diseases) and other essential nutrients, and tends to crowd them out of your diet. It is now proven that consuming too much meat can lead to colon, prostate and breast cancer.

Sugar

You may think that sugar gives you energy but in fact it is an energy sapper. Sugar floods the bloodstream giving you an instant but brief high. Once the high has subsided your energy levels drop lower than they were to start with. Refined sugars – which these days are to be found in everything from cornflakes to gherkins – also contribute to poor skin as the safest place for toxins to overflow is through the pores. Keep an eye on food labels and watch out for high sugar content or chemical sugar replacements. Most ingredients ending with the letters '-ose' contain high quantities of sugar. Food labels now tell you what proportion of the carbohydrate content is made up of sugars.

Heather: *I remember my husband telling me a story about how he visited a sugar refinery in Cuba. The first vat he came to, molasses, smelt delicious. The second, of brown sugar, smelt even sweeter. But the third smelt foul. 'What's that dreadful smell?' he asked. 'Oh that,' they said. 'That's for you foreigners. We put bleach in that because you crazy guys like it white.'*

Salt

Our bodies need salt, for one thing it has a large part to play in regulating your body's fluid balance. You should be able to get all the salt you need if you eat plenty of fresh vegetables. You do not need to pour table salt all over everything you eat. Excessive salt intake stimulates the adrenal glands so leading to stress arousal, high blood pressure and all the problems associated with it such as increased risk of stroke, heart failure and kidney failure.

Salt is often used as a 'natural' preservative. Eliminating

or cutting down on processed foods is one of the best ways to reduce your salt intake. Other ways to cut down include not adding salt at the table (taste your food before adding salt, don't just add it out of habit), substituting unsalted nuts and raw vegetables for crisps and salted nuts, and rinsing olives, pickles and sauerkraut before serving them.

Caffeine

Caffeine in coffee, tea and many colas and soft drinks boosts the body's output of stress hormones. The immediate effect is to make us feel more alert but before long this gives way to irritability, muscular fatigue and lethargy. Great alternatives are decaffeinated coffee, green tea and white tea. Buy the organic brands as organic coffee processing uses water filtration rather than chemicals – the chemicals used for non-organic coffee processing often end up in your cup. Green tea contains small amounts of caffeine but also powerful antioxidants which protect the heart and arteries against oxidative damage and may reduce the risk of cancer. White tea contains the same antioxidants but a low amount of caffeine. Some people find the taste a bit overpowering (and you don't need to add milk). Drink it weak at first. If you are a confirmed tea or coffee drinker you will get withdrawal symptoms such as headaches if you stop drinking them suddenly. This should give you a clue as to their not being particularly good for you. Cut down gradually.

Additives

Additives are nearly all chemically-derived and as such they add to the amount of toxic waste which the body has to deal with. They include colourings, flavourings, sweeteners, preservatives, antioxidants, stabilizers, emulsifiers and modi-fied starches. Some food manufacturers use up to 100 chemicals to produce just one flavour. Read labels and avoid additives.

Weight Loss

There are no miracle cures for being overweight. The common sense advice given by most doctors to anyone who wants to achieve and maintain their optimum weight is simple: eat a healthy diet and take regular exercise. There really is no quick fix.

You should never underestimate the power of a bad slimming diet to make you feel miserable! It is often believed that for food to be good for you it can't be enjoyable. This is nonsense. Any healthy-eating plan which eliminates real pleasure is almost certain to fail. Bear in mind, though, that fat accounts for much of the flavour of food. For many people the pleasure derived from eating will drop con-siderably once the fat content drops to 20% or less of the total intake. Most people can enjoy good health on a diet containing 30% fat and the traditional Mediterranean diet suggests that in some circumstances even more fat in the diet might be acceptable. There are good and bad fats. Avoid all processed trans fats, they clog your arteries and can lead to many health problems. Avoid, where possible, hydrogenated fats and minimize saturated fats to 2g per serving. Polyunsaturated and mono-unsaturated are the good fats your body needs to protect muscle tissues and fibres. You can work out the percentage fat content by reading the labels on your food, usually the fat content per 100g is given. By the way, traditional Oriental diets have a fat content of only about 10%, the delicious flavours being derived from subtle herbs and spices.

Reading Labels

There are people who take the complexities of label reading on food packaging very seriously but a few basic rules of thumb are all that are needed. Note the fat and sugar content; avoid products that contain artificial additives (colourings, flavourings, sweeteners, preservatives, antioxidants, stabilizers, emulsifiers and modified starches); avoid products with very long lists of ingredients; and avoid products which contain ingredients you can't pronounce!

Statements such as 'low fat' or even 'fat free' do not necessarily mean that a product is slimming. If manufacturers remove fat from, say, biscuits, they replace the fat with more sugar in order to boost the flavour. Terms such as 'lite' and 'extra lite' are meaningless. This often just means that there is a smaller quantity of the product in the packet. If something is 90% fat free it still contains 10% pure fat – and that can mean a lot of fat.

Also watch out for 'no added sugar'. This doesn't mean that the food is sugar-free, it means that sugar hasn't been added generally because the product already has a naturally high sugar content.

When to Eat

Heather: *I generally have a big breakfast, a medium lunch and a light dinner. We're all wired differently and this happens* *to work best for me. I always carry a bottle of water and some nibbles with me when I travel – things like raisins, nuts, rice cakes, tofu chunks, fruit salad, bananas, sunflower seeds or apples. I enjoy snacking throughout the day so it's very important that I always have a proper supply of healthy snacks. If I don't, I am tempted to eat the first thing that comes to hand which, when I'm travelling, is likely to be junk food.*

If you eat three meals a day you may find your blood sugar levels decline between meals. This is why so many of us feel drowsy mid-afternoon.

A healthy, low-sugar, slow energy release snack such as sunflower seeds will stave off any hunger pangs mid-morning and mid-afternoon and help keep your energy at a constant level. A final snack before bed is okay as long as you avoid eating anything too heavy and you stay clear of stimulants such as caffeine, cheese or chocolate.

Vital Energy

A meal's nourishing quality does not only come from the food itself. Preparing and eating the most basic of meals can be pleasurable if you approach it in the right way. Food contains something more than the sum of its ingredients. Immerse yourself in the process of preparing and eating food so that the task itself becomes a form of meditation. Try to savour every second of preparation, every bite of food. Take the same care in the preparation of food when you are on your own as you would cooking for other people. It may take a little longer to prepare and eat a meal and to clean up afterwards – washing up is a wonderful meditation practice –

but the 'mindfulness' of food can be just as conducive to well-being as the nutrients are beneficial to the body.

The Optimum Diet

To summarize, the principles behind an optimum diet are simple:

1. **Give your body the nutrients it needs**. Eat plenty of good quality, fresh vegetables, whole grains, pulses and fruit.
2. **Avoid negative or harmful foodstuffs**. Try not to eat foods which are bad for you, or which cause suffering to others or damage the environment. You'll do best to avoid animal fats altogether and be careful to take only small quantities of salt, refined and processed foods and additives. Also try to keep a watchful eye on your intake of wheat. If possible buy only organic products and drink plenty of distilled or purified water.
3. **Enjoy!** Remember that planning, preparing and cooking a meal can be every bit as pleasurable as the meal itself.

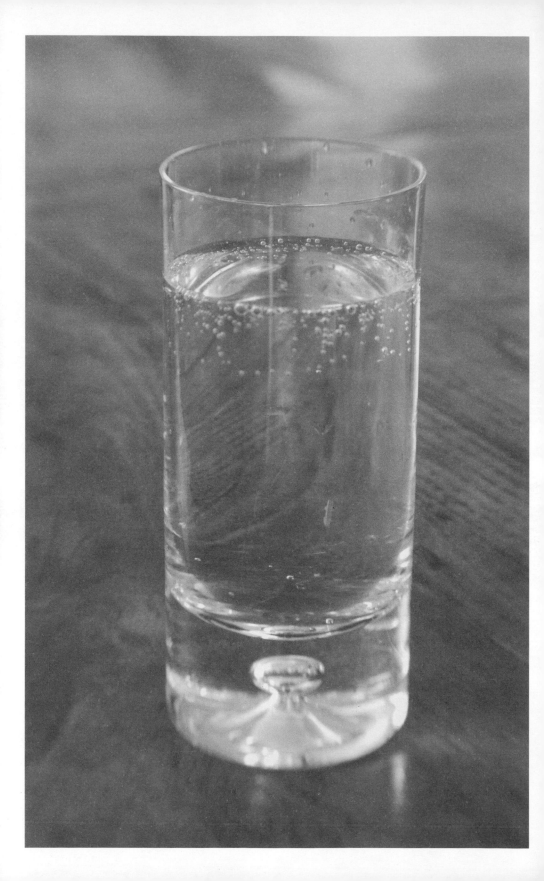

10 | Detoxing Your Body

Heather: *I try to detox my body periodically to clear out any toxins from my system. I eat a balanced and healthy diet now so detoxing isn't as tough as it used to be when my diet was awful and my body responded strongly to being deprived of the chemicals and pollutants which are present in so many modern foodstuffs. I once coincided a detox with a time when I had a lot of meetings scheduled. Add to that the fact that it was during the cold and dark of winter and I can now appreciate why I found that particular detox extremely gruelling – I just wanted to curl up and nurture myself with food. Since then I've been more careful to choose the right moment. I find a good time to start is when I'm on a summer holiday. The last time I did a juice fast like the one we show you in this chapter was when I was on a Caribbean holiday. It was difficult because there was so much delicious food about but my energy levels were so great by the morning of the third day that, although I did go back to eating solid food, I didn't really want to!*

Ben: *Heather taught me a valuable trick – when I start a detox I clear out cupboards and the fridge of food that's bad for me and*

139

I turn the TV on to another channel when commercials begin. I really don't want to watch someone in a state of ecstasy eating a cream cheese bagel or a chocolate bar when I'm valiantly sipping spring water! I also avoid dinner parties during the first week. It's a good idea to read this chapter all the way through before undertaking a detox so you know just what to expect. For instance, your body will tell you that it needs more food when in fact it is simply craving toxins so don't be misled by these signals. Paradoxically, feeling bad during a detox is a good sign. Prepare yourself for the fact that altering your eating habits, even for a short period, can be pretty tough!

Always check with your doctor first before undertaking any detox routine.

The detox regime we find helpful begins with a pre-detox week followed by a weekend juice fast, a few days of readjustment, and four weeks of eating sensibly. Six weeks may seem a lot of time to commit to a detox regime but remember that only one week – the juice fast and readjustment – requires any real discipline. The rest of the time you are simply eating well and avoiding taking in any more toxins.

Pre-Detox Week

Begin with a little self-assessment. How much alcohol, tea or coffee do you consume during the course of a week? How much bottled or filtered water do you drink? How many portions of fruit or fresh, raw vegetables do you eat? Make a note in your notebook of your intake of less healthy foods such as animal fats, additives and sugar. It is a good way to remind yourself of the foods you most want to avoid throughout the detox period and makes interesting reading after you've finished!

During the pre-detox week cut down tea or coffee to a maximum of one cup a day. Increase your fruit and veg portions to two each per day. Drink several glasses of bottled or filtered water daily. Significantly reduce your intake of wheat, dairy products, animal fats, sugar, salt, additives and refined or processed foods.

Some people choose to undergo colonic irrigation during this week as it is an ideal time to do it. The narrowing of the colonic lining caused by the build-up of waste deposits stops essential minerals and vitamins from being efficiently absorbed into the body. Animal protein in particular can clog the bowel – it can sometimes stay in the colon for years. Colonic irrigation clears away waste to allow essential vitamins and minerals to be absorbed along the densely vascular lining of the colon and also allows toxic waste to be propelled more effectively towards the rectum and discharged from the body.

Colonic irrigation is sometimes considered dangerous or unnatural but when it is performed by a trained practitioner there is no reason why it should be in any way harmful. A colonic therapy session may leave you feeling tired for a day or two afterwards if you are very toxic so make sure you don't have the treatment when you're very busy.

Heather: *When I was in hospital for three months after my accident, I became so constipated as a result of the hospital diet and all the medication that I did not have a bowel movement during the whole time. One of my injuries was a crushed pelvis – more painful than losing my leg. A friend suggested a colonic,*

141

which I'd never heard of, but I was willing to try anything. Six pounds of waste later, I was on cloud nine and my pain was greatly diminished. The waste had been pressing on my broken pelvis. I think colonics in ill health or constipation are incredible. I have heard it said that they 'wash away the good bacteria,' but just try and find any good bacteria in a mound of constipated, poisonous bowel waste and gases! If you have a healthy lifestyle you won't need a colonic.

Juice Fast Weekend

During the juice fast weekend you will not be eating any solids. Instead, your diet will consist of vegetable or fruit juices. This two-day juice fast really kick-starts the detox process. Juicing causes your blood sugar levels to rise sharply so if you suffer from low blood sugar, candida or diabetes skip this stage and move straight to the Readjustment Days.

Make your juice from any vegetables you like or from non-acidic fruits such as apples and pears. Dilute the juice 50:50 with bottled or filtered water and drink plenty of water between juices to further cleanse your system.

You are bound to be hungry and a little tired during these two days. Resist the temptation to eat any solids but if hunger really gets the better of you have a few seedless grapes.

Epsom salts can be great for drawing toxins out of the skin, so pamper yourself with lots of Epsom salt baths throughout the detox. Pour a couple of cups of Epsom salts into a blood-heat bath. Epsom salts are a good way of counteracting the bloating and wind that are inevitable side effects of cleansing your body. Remember, there are plenty of ways to pamper yourself without gorging on food so really go to town during a detox.

Readjustment Days

By the beginning of day three your body will have started to adjust and you can begin to reintroduce food to your diet. For the rest of the week continue the readjustment process by eating as many vegetables, whole grains and non-acidic fruit and drinking as much filtered or bottled water as you want. This means avoiding the following:

additives
alcohol
animal fats
avocados
bananas (these can be quite difficult to digest post-detox)
bread
caffeine
chocolate
dairy products
eggs
fish
lentils (these can create excess wind, and you've probably
   had enough of that already!)
mushrooms (if you suffer from candida you might want to
   avoid these for a while)
oranges
pasta
peanuts
refined or processed foods

salt
spinach
sugar
tomatoes (these are very acidic)
wheat

This is a detox, not a slimming diet, so if you feel hungry eat something – but not something from the above list.

Try to eat organic food only, because you are ridding yourself of the harmful toxins present in almost all non-organic produce. Organic produce is superior to non-organic foods in that it is free from toxins and pollutants. Raw vegetables are superior to cooked vegetables because they have retained their nutrients. The closer food comes to its natural state and the closer it is to its raw form, the higher is its quality or 'life force'.

Weeks 2–5

For the following four weeks continue to eat plenty of fresh, raw or almost-raw vegetables and non-acidic fruit; drink plenty of bottled or filtered water; cut out all stimulants such as caffeine, sugar and alcohol; and cut back on carbohydrates other than cereals and whole grains. Take home-prepared containers of food to work with you if necessary, to avoid the temptations of the sandwich bar, and be careful to stick to detox foods when eating out.

What to Expect

You are likely to experience some side effects when undergoing a detox. Just knowing what to expect can help. The more sleep or rest you have the more quickly any symptoms will disappear. Allow yourself plenty of time to rest and go easy on yourself during this period. Keep on reminding yourself of the long-term benefits, and stick with it.

Tiredness

The human body tends towards optimum health: broken bones heal, torn tissues reconstruct themselves, germs are expelled. In the same way your body will discard lower-grade tissues and materials if superior tissues are available. When you improve the quality of the food you eat your body will immediately set about breaking down inferior body tissue and replacing it with higher-grade material. Your energy levels are likely to take a temporary dip as a result of this process. Don't worry, they will come back up again.

During a detox you are abandoning ingredients such as salt, sugar and spices, all of which are stimulants. Without these stimulants the action of the heart decreases a little which also contributes to a drop in energy levels. Irritants such as food preservatives, aspirins and drugs are expelled from the body as are fat masses, sludge from the arteries, bile from the gall bladder and liver and arthritic deposits from the joints. The whole lot is broken down and removed, a process which requires quite a lot of physical energy. During this process your body redeploys energy from other places such as from muscle movement – the brain sends out a message to your muscles ordering them to slow down and relax, in the form of tiredness.

 This period of lethargy generally lasts for a few weeks during which time you should listen to what your body is telling you and take it easy. Don't give in to the temptation to revert to your old ways: if you stick with it, after just a few short weeks your energy levels will be significantly greater than before you began the detox. What's more, they should stay there. The poor quality of the foods we generally take in means that few things have so profound an effect on our vibrancy and energy levels as improving how we eat.

Weight changes

You may experience some weight loss as body tissue is broken down and removed. When the excess of obstructing material in the tissues has been eliminated, your body weight will stabilize for a while before going up again temporarily. This is entirely normal. Despite the fact that you are taking in fewer calories there is no longer any low-quality tissue to be discarded and the new, better-quality tissues do not break down so easily. Your body's improved assimilation means that new tissues are now being formed faster and your body requires less food as a result. This doesn't always tally with the habits of a lifetime! Your weight will soon stabilize and you may well find that you want to eat smaller portions than before your detox.

Skin problems

One of the ways in which the human body discards toxins is through the skin. If you find that your complexion is not as good as normal, remind yourself that having a few weeks of less than beautiful skin is a small price to pay for good health. Better out than in. In a very short time any breakouts will clear and you should find that your skin is glowing with good health.

Cold symptoms

As your body continues to houseclean you might also develop a cold. Don't try to counteract these symptoms with drugs or doses of vitamins as this is tantamount to attempting to cure a cure. Your body is healing itself, so let it.

Headaches and digestive discomfort

Other possible side effects of a full detox include headaches, irritability, bowel sluggishness and frequent urination or diarrhoea. It is unlikely that you will get more than one or two of these and only for a short period. If you bear in mind why they are happening it will make them easier to cope with. These are the wastes which might otherwise, if trapped in the body, have brought you long-term pain or disease. The more difficult the side effects you experience during your detox the greater the potential illness, pain or suffering your body might otherwise have succumbed to.

Headaches and irritability are the most common side effects that people experience on a detox. Here is a quick exercise that can help:

Sit down, make yourself comfortable and take 20 very deep breaths into your belly. Don't forget the final 'top-up' of breath as that is where the magic of a breathing detox happens.

After nine or ten breaths you should begin to enjoy a feeling of serenity and well-being coming over you. By the time you reach 20 notice how clear-headed you feel. The chances are you are at least 50% calmer than you were a few moments ago when you began.

Many people find that they rush a little during the first few breaths, impatient to get the exercise over with. If this is how you respond you can take this as a clear sign that the pace of your life is too frantic at the moment and you could benefit from slowing down a little.

Overall you can expect a pattern of three steps forward and one step back. You will begin to feel progressively better then you may feel a little nauseous for a day. You will then feel even better than before followed perhaps by a day of diarrhoea. You recover and go even higher, and then another reaction occurs and you don't feel so well again. Each setback is milder than the last and each period of feeling better lasts longer. Soon you will reach a plateau of health and vibrancy and you will feel better and more energized than you have done for years.

Who wouldn't exchange a few weeks of feeling a little under par for a lifetime of increased energy and vibrancy?

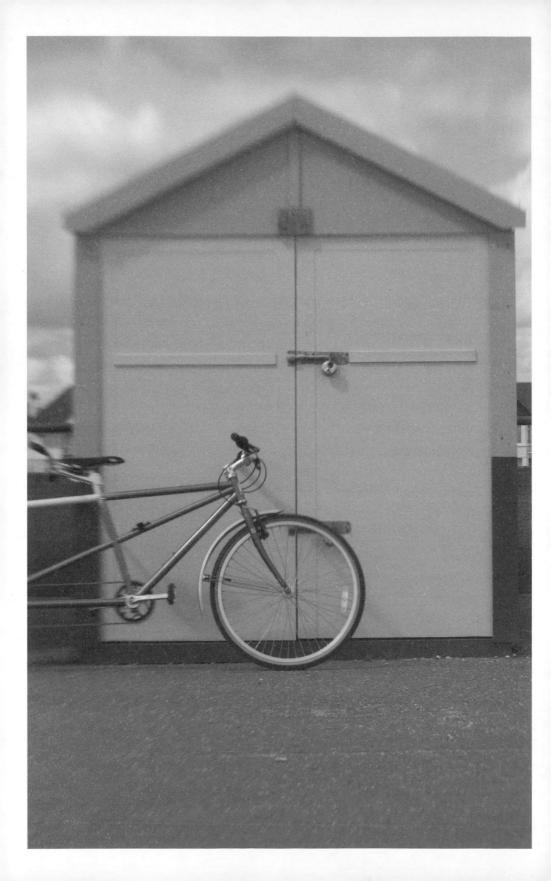

11 | Exercise

Heather: *My father was a pentathlete and wanted to live out his dreams through his children. He was very encouraging on the exercise front when I was younger, perhaps too much so. My sister did synchronized swimming, my brother did a bit of sports, and I was very much into athletics and swimming. I was in it for the medals, pure and simple. I took sport very seriously. For quite a long time I used to get up each morning at 6 a.m. and make my way down to the gym. In retrospect I can see that I exercised too much.*

These days at the gym I focus on weight training as well as Pilates and yoga, and I'll also do a few squats and exercises for my leg. If I don't exercise my leg I risk getting atrophy where the limb begins to waste away. I try to take regular exercise because of the significant effect it has on my health and well-being.

Ben: *The amount of feel-good that can result from just a small amount of exercise is amazing. It needn't be expensive and it can be done almost whenever, wherever. Heather and I joined a gym in North London when we shared an office. The difference between us was that Heather actually visited it. Heather used to shout across the office to me that I needed to go to the gym, but*

I feigned deafness. Going to the gym just isn't my thing. What I prefer – and how I now get my exercise – is long, easy walks across Hampstead Heath with Harvey, my Springer Spaniel. I love walking. It doesn't lead to a release of endorphins so I don't feel the 'high' which many people chase after in the gym, but I find a real degree of serenity on my walks.

Heather: *My personality type is fairly addictive – I can be a person of extremes. I have learnt that this can be very positive when properly channelled but I need to be careful about overdoing anything, particularly exercise. You can get addicted to the 'happy drugs' the body produces during exercise.* **Moderate** *exercise is one of the most positive things you can introduce into your life. There is always an opportunity to take exercise, no matter where you are. Even if I'm spending the day sitting on an aeroplane on a long-haul flight, I'll still get a small workout together by walking up and down the aisles and tensing my bum muscles. And no, I don't really care what people think, after all, it's my body!*

Exercise is without doubt one of the best things you can do for yourself. Not only does it make you look and feel better, it also improves the quality of your sleep, lowers stress levels and sharpens your concentration. Exercise enhances self-esteem, relieves depression and frustration, reduces weight and increases energy levels. By anyone's standards this is impressive stuff! Add to this the fact that remaining physically fit reduces the risk of premature death by an astonishing 40%, and the case for incorporating regular exercise into your daily routine becomes overwhelming.

Until relatively recently our ancestors planted and harvested crops, chopped wood, scrubbed floors and washed clothes by hand. The wonders of modern technology mean that today more than 60% of the adult population isn't regularly active and 25% is scarcely active at all. The average American watches three and a half hours of television daily, time which a century ago would have been spent doing manual chores. Humans are physiologically predisposed to exercise regularly yet most of us don't.

There is one overwhelming reason why people don't exercise – it is too much effort. The word 'exercise' is itself enough to send cold shivers down many people's spines. Taking exercise can be a lot of fun, especially when you begin to feel and see the results. It is not long before you stop associating exercise with pain, sweat and tight clothes which pronounce every unsightly bulge, and start thinking instead of the amazing benefits. If you're one of life's couch potatoes listen up: if you really want to look and feel good, regular exercise isn't optional, it's essential.

A Natural High

There is another reason why people take regular exercise: **they enjoy it!**

During exercise your body releases feel-good chemicals – endorphins, serotonin, adrenalin and dopamine. Endorphins are the brain's painkillers and are three times more powerful than morphine. Serotonin helps maintain a feeling of happiness. Adrenalin keeps you alert. One of the side effects of dopamine is that it reduces the desire to overeat. After taking even moderate amounts of exercise, therefore, you will start to feel good. Exercise is a great way to achieve a natural high.

There are other potential benefits too, such as better sex. A toned and fit body is definitely sexy, which is just as well as many people report an increased sex drive after taking up regular exercise. These people also noticed their sex life was more vigorous but that wasn't a problem either because they were more flexible and had increased stamina as a result of taking regular exercise. Increased levels of certain brain chemicals released during exercise can also make sex more pleasurable.

If this has finally sold the idea of exercise to you there are a few things you should bear in mind ...

Be Safe

Anyone can take up exercise, young or old, but if you are in any doubt about your health consult your GP before embarking on a fitness regime. **Don't** exercise if you are unwell, in pain from an injury, you have taken drugs or alcohol or have eaten a heavy meal, if you have taken painkillers (they will mask any warning signs), or if you are undergoing medical treatment.

The right equipment
Getting kitted out properly is essential. Make sure the shoes you wear are appropriate for your chosen activity. There is little point in taking up exercise if you're wearing a pair of old plimsolls dug out of a box in the attic as the damage done to your joints will outweigh any of the health benefits. This doesn't mean you have to spend a fortune on kit: a decent pair of trainers can be bought for around £40.

Exercise

Warm-up/cool-down

Incorporate a warm-up and cool-down session into any exercise routine. Gently stretch your muscles and increase your respiration, circulation and body temperature before you start, and decrease them with some low impact exercises before you finish. This will add just three to five minutes to your routine and will help prevent injury.

A good warm-up/cool-down exercise is to stand upright with your feet together. Take a step forward with your left foot. Slightly bend your left knee while keeping your right heel on the ground and your right leg straight. Hold this position for a few seconds – you should feel a mild stretch around the calf muscle on your right leg. Stand with your feet together again and repeat the exercise for the other leg. At the end of your exercise session also spend a few minutes walking slowly and stretching to prevent your muscles from feeling tight and uncomfortable. A cool-down routine also brings down your heart rate.

Don't overdo it

Exercise gives you a buzz that can last for several days. As the buzz subsides you may feel compelled to exercise even more vigorously to keep your 'happy high' topped up. When you overdo exercise the chemicals which previously led to a feeling of well-being can instead cause feelings of anxiety, anger or irritation – the very things that a moderate exercise routine burns off. So take it easy! Don't try to do too much too soon. 'No pain, no gain' is a myth. The key to exercising properly is moderation.

Eat well

For most people being overweight is evidence that they are not successfully balancing their energy input (food) and output (exercise), and doctors agree that by eating sensibly and taking regular exercise most people will not get overweight. But that's like a non-smoker thinking that a smoker simply has to stop smoking. It's not that easy. Eating well and taking regular exercise requires a lifestyle choice and plenty of willpower. But the payback is wonderful.

Once you start exercising you will burn more calories and you will need to eat more and better food. It is no good gorging yourself on fast food or chocolate, you need to feed yourself with good, healthy food. Complex carbohydrates such as pasta and wholemeal bread release energy slowly over a period of hours and they will help give you stamina and energy. Bananas and dried fruits are a good source of sugar and preferable to chocolate or sweets. Take a little time to discover which healthy foods you enjoy.

Be Balanced

Find a form of exercise that suits you. If you don't like it then you won't stay with it, it's as simple as that. If you don't think of yourself as a sporty person at all you are probably wasting your time squeezing yourself into a lycra body suit and heading down to the gym. Perhaps you would be temperamentally better suited to walking to and from work, or taking up cycling or dancing.

There are two types of exercise: aerobic and anaerobic. **Aerobic** exercise (literally meaning 'air-life') keeps your heart and lungs healthy. It is low in intensity but long in duration, such as brisk walking, jogging, cycling, swimming or dancing. It is a great way to get into shape if you haven't taken any exercise for a while. **Anaerobic** exercise emphasizes endurance and building muscle, for example, weight training.

The human body needs both aerobic and anaerobic exercise and the best exercise routine therefore combines both, such as power walking or jogging with a sprint finish. Or you can vary your exercise routine with a walk one day and weight training the next.

Weights

Some women are a bit wary of weight training, thinking that it might give them big muscles. The opposite is true. Muscle development depends on the hormone testosterone and women have only one-tenth the amount of testosterone as men. Of course, if you pump iron for five hours a day for a year you may start looking like Popeye, but this is not something which will happen without a huge amount of effort on your part! As with most things, moderation is the key. The great thing about gaining muscle over fat is that you end up burning calories at rest – doing absolutely nothing. Join a gym and explain to the instructor what it is you are trying to achieve.

Jogging

Perhaps the easiest form of exercise is donning a tracksuit and jogging around the block. With jogging you are not depending on anyone else to make you take exercise (if your golfing or tennis partner can't make it then neither can you), and you can modify the length of your jog according to your mood or circumstances. Listen to music while you jog to keep you company. You don't have to jog on your own street or on busy roads. Find somewhere pleasant – a park or a nice quiet street – even if you have to hop on a bus or drive a few miles to get there.

Swimming

Jogging can be harsh on your joints and for this reason many doctors recommend swimming as an alternative. Swimming works on the upper and lower body rather than concentrating almost exclusively on the legs. An obvious difficulty with taking up swimming is that you have to schedule in the journey time to and from the pool. Having to find an additional 45 minutes or hour for travelling could make all the difference between exercising daily or not at all.

The gym

The same is true with joining a gym. Having paid a membership fee most people feel that they will be more likely to continue going once the novelty has worn off. The reality is somewhat different, many people join their local gyms only to stop going after the first few weeks. Joining a gym does have great advantages, particularly that your fitness programme can be drawn up and regulated by a qualified trainer. Most gyms offer an initial appraisal for free upon joining from which they can advise you as to the best form of exercise for your needs and preferences, such as circuit training, swimming or running. Many gyms also have a crèche.

Some gyms offer team sports such as tennis, soccer or squash. Team sports have the advantage that you may feel compelled to don your trainers because you have made a commitment to other people, even on days when you are lacking motivation. They can also be a lot of fun as long as the competitive spirit doesn't become too important and you and your partners or opponents agree as to whether you are playing for fun and fitness or playing to win. So be sure to establish your respective objectives from the outset!

Pilates

Pilates is a system of exercise which draws on skiing, yoga, gymnastics, dance, circus training and weight training to give the body a perfect balance of strength and flexibility. Pilates is a fairly gentle form of exercise, more like yoga than aerobics. It is as much about opening and expanding the mind as it is about physical fitness and is widely recognized as a good antidote to stress and anxiety. It is also seen as highly effective for the elderly and for rehabilitation after illness, because its gentle exercises involve little muscular stress, and no jumping or bouncing around. Pilates is said to prevent injury; it can lead to increased mobility in the joints and improved circulation; and its emphasis upon correct posture means that it can also benefit people who suffer from arthritis and osteoporosis.

It is not an activity just for the elderly or the infirm – far from it! Pilates is recognized as one of the most effective means of reducing tummy bulges. It is ideal for women who want to regain their shape after pregnancy as well as those people who simply want to stay in great shape.

The Pilates Method was developed in the early part of the twentieth century by Joseph H. Pilates. At the outbreak of the First World War, as a German living in England, Joseph was interned for the duration. He used this time to develop a series of exercises which he taught to fellow detainees. After the war he set up a fitness studio in New York where he taught his technique to an assortment of willing volunteers, from boxers to members of the New York City Ballet. Joseph Pilates died in a fire at his studio in 1967, never having laid down a precise method of body conditioning. In the subsequent decades his core techniques have been developed and expanded upon by a number of teachers. As a result there are any number of Pilates schools and practices, all of them based upon the general teachings of the founder but each unique in its own way.

If you are going to take up exercise after a long period of inactivity you could do worse than begin with Pilates. A wide variety of books and tapes are readily available and, because Pilates has become almost as popular as yoga in recent years, classes are now commonplace. See the internet, your local library or community notice board for further information.

Life as your gym

You can still incorporate exercise into your everyday life even if you can't find a sport or exercise you like. Climb the stairs rather than using the lift, park your car in the farthest spot in the car park, or cycle to work. The drawback with this sort of exercise, of course, is that there are countless labour-saving devices within arm's reach to entice you away from your new-found resolutions. 'Why should I walk to the shops when I can drive?' 'Why use the stairs when there's a lift?' All it takes is an 'off' day and you may find your old habits returning for good.

Use your imagination. The next time the kids step out of the house for 20 minutes put on some music and try dancing. You may feel a bit daft at first but who cares? No one can see you. Exercise videos can be great, too, especially if you work out with a friend. Remember that this is **your** exercise routine and keep to it even if your partner can't make it. Exercise shouldn't be a chore. Keep looking and you're likely to find an activity you like.

Make a Commitment

Once you have chosen your activity, whether it is working out at the gym or simply a lunchtime walk in the park, make a commitment to it. Write down when you are going to begin exercising – the time, the place – and stick to it!

Exercise at a time of the day which suits **you**. If you have a shower and somewhere to change at work, why not jog or cycle to and from the office? Lunchtime is also a good time to exercise, but not on a full stomach. As a rule it's not a good idea to exercise shortly before bedtime as your body will be full of energizing 'happy drugs' and you may feel too 'buzzy' to sleep.

One of the main reasons people give up exercise is over-doing it in the first few weeks. Just five or ten minutes every other day for the first two or three weeks should be ample, gradually increasing throughout the first month or two until you are exercising most days for 15 minutes or so. As a general rule, a short workout most days is preferable to a long workout once a fortnight.

The benefits of a low-intensity exercise routine are difficult to exaggerate. If you don't have time to exercise, make the time. There are 168 hours in a week. A 15-minute daily exercise routine adds up to less than two hours a week. This is something which almost anyone can achieve. Most people set aside at least six times as long as this for eating. It is all a matter of whether you want to look and feel great.

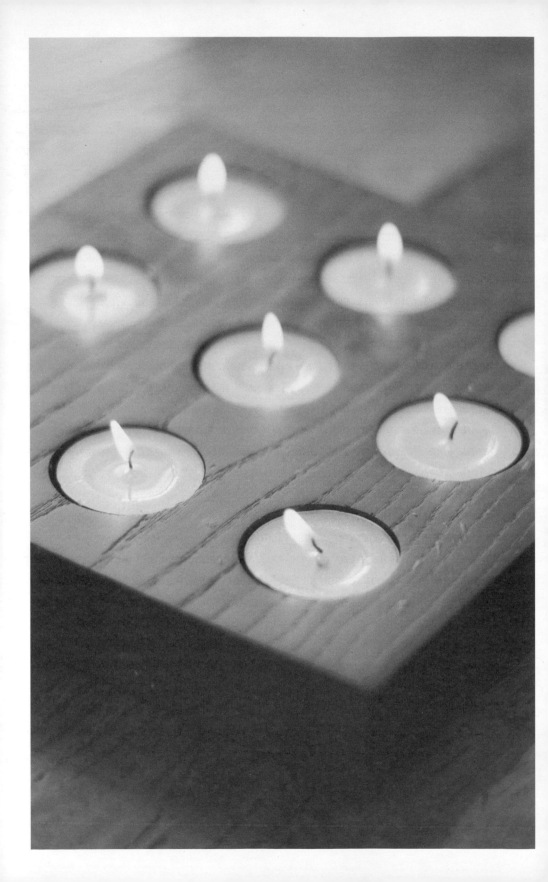

12 | Yoga

Heather: *A few years ago Paul and I went to Rajistan. While we were there we met the most amazing yoga teacher. He was an incredible person, radiating joy and serenity with every movement and from every pore. His body was slim and well toned and he could put his legs behind his head without any difficulty. There wouldn't have been anything particularly remarkable about this, except that he was in his eighties! Exceptional people like this are to be found all over the East but they are comparatively rare in Europe – at least, I've yet to meet an 85-year-old Londoner with anything like this sort of flexibility. The secret is simple: yoga.*

Since the birth of our daughter I have become aware of how supple and flexible human beings are when they are born. And there is no real reason for us to lose that flexibility. Two of the key signs of ageing are reduced movement and loss of good posture, yet there's no reason why we should stoop or dodder as middle age creeps in. Certainly, I have no intention of creaking my way through life. Yoga is concerned with how you feel rather than with outward appearances but an inevitable consequence of feeling great is that you look great, too.

Ben: *Although I'm fairly fit and flexible, yoga didn't come easily to me and one of the first things I had to overcome was the need to compete with other people in the class. I also had to overcome the desire to howl with laughter when people started snoring during the relaxation or 'Corpse Position'! But I'm glad I persevered: I am more relaxed and easier to get on with in daily life when I'm regularly practising yoga, and some long-term aches and pains have improved a great deal. They say that yoga makes you look better, feel younger and stay connected. Although these sound like extravagant promises, broadly speaking I believe them to be true.*

Yoga serves as a powerful link between physical disciplines like exercise and more spiritual pursuits such as meditation. It is a unifying bond between the physical and spiritual aspects of ourselves and it plays a crucial role in our well-being. The West is centuries behind Eastern philosophy when it comes to recognizing the significant importance of equilibrium in our lives.

Yoga first appeared in India around 5000 years ago. The word **yoga** derives from the Sanskrit word 'yug', meaning 'to yoke' or 'join together'. In general terms it means joining the physical and the emotional, body and mind. In spiritual terms it refers to the union of the individual consciousness to the universal consciousness. Yoga is much more than a practice for mind/body balance – its goal is spiritual enlightenment.

Many types of yoga have emerged over its long history, including Hatha, Karma, Kriya, Raja, Bakti, Tantra, Mantra and Jnana yoga. Some people have tunnel vision about particular schools but each has its own worth and there are some basic principles that are common to almost all schools of yoga. This is what we will be looking at in this section.

You don't have to be in the least bit spiritual to take up yoga. Anyone can practise it, regardless of age or belief. It is not a religion and many of yoga's millions of adherents practise it entirely for practical reasons. Yoga has the effect of stretching and toning, increasing lung capacity, alleviating tiredness, improving flexibility and mobility, easing back pain and improving heart conditions. It makes you feel good and there can be no better reason to take it up than that. Several progressive insurance companies now include yoga in their alternative therapies coverage and it is not difficult to see why. Any doctor will tell you that moderate exercise, deep breathing and relaxation are great ways to alleviate stress. Practitioners of yoga tend to be less anxious, less dependent on external factors for happiness, and less adversely affected by life's difficulties and disappointments than non-practitioners.

Aspects of Yoga

Many people in the West prefer to concentrate on the purely practical benefits of yoga. That's fine, but it does miss the point. It's a bit like buying a state of the art laptop and only using it for writing memos. Yoga has so much more to offer than stretching and flexing.

Traditional yoga has three aspects: body control, breath control and mind control. The postures (**asanas**) keep the body stress-free; the breathing exercises (**pranayama**) keep the mind stress-free; and the combination of the two enables the practitioner to experience a meditative state in which the mind is brought towards equilibrium (**samadhi**). The key to yoga's potency is this synthesis of your whole being – body, mind and spirit. Yoga has been described as something which happens **to** you. It exercises the body, mind and spirit all together.

The true yogi, by tradition, follows a path of loving kindness devoid of violence, greed or deceit. The fact that so many people in the West question the relevance of this aspect of yoga, or dismiss it entirely, says a lot more about us than it does about the yogic tradition. The practical benefits of yoga are no more than pleasing by-products of this ancient and sacred practice. If yoga were useful for toning and stretching and nothing more than that, it probably would not have endured down the ages.

Yoga and Your Body

Whatever your approach to yoga you cannot avoid being toned and honed by its exercises. When you first take up yoga you may discover muscles you never knew you had and you should also notice a marked improvement in your breathing and in your posture. Yoga addresses areas of your body which are overlooked by conventional exercise and because of this it effectively complements other forms of exercise. For instance, most joggers have shallow breathing patterns. Yoga's deep breathing exercises increase the flow of oxygen to the brain and improve a runner's endurance. Yoga also strengthens joints such as hips, feet, knees and ankles, all of which are put under pressure when jogging. Flexible joggers are less likely to sustain an injury. Swimmers, too, benefit from the increased strength and flexibility that come with regular yoga practice, and from the added control they have over their breathing.

It is also beneficial for people using weights – yoga lengthens the muscles which are built up during weight training and keeps them flexible. It makes breathing and balance easier while working out. Yoga itself is a form of weightlifting, with your body being the weights.

Choosing a Class

It is far easier to master the processes of yoga in a class where you have an instructor to guide you. Furthermore, you are less likely to skip a yoga session if you are a paid-up member of a group meeting at specific times and you may find that the company inspires you and sustains your interest. You will also benefit from having an instructor on hand who can advise you with regard to specific problems you may have such as back pain. And if you are pregnant, always check with your GP before taking up a new form of exercise.

There are two things to remember when finding a class to join:

1. Anyone can set up a yoga class, you don't need to be a qualified instructor. Make sure that the instructor really knows what they are talking about.
2. Make sure that your instructor shares your own vision of what you want to achieve. If you are interested in mind–body–spirit balance as practised in traditional yoga, don't join a 'yoga-cise' class where the objective is to stretch and tone.

Try out a single session before enrolling for the entire series. Even a qualified instructor might be a poor teacher!

There will generally be a choice of several classes in most towns or cities so don't feel committed to the first one you look at. You can get details of classes from health clubs, fitness stores, health food stores, local libraries, community colleges or from the internet. Try to find a class which is small so you get plenty of individual attention. If you can't get to a yoga class or you prefer to work alone, there are several excellent yoga videos available. Some people prefer audio tapes as you don't have to keep glancing at the TV screen. Most large lending libraries have yoga videos and audio tapes.

Getting Started

We strongly recommend that you learn a couple of basic postures before joining a group, such as the Mountain Pose (below). This may seem the wrong way around but even the most basic beginners' class is usually a mixture of 'Level 2' exercises – standing, sitting and lying poses – whereas it is a good idea to get the hang of the most **basic** standing poses before moving on to sitting or lying positions.

Spend a few minutes each day practising. Set aside a regular time for your session and for the first couple of weeks keep your sessions to between ten and fifteen minutes each: two or three minutes for warming up, five to ten minutes of yoga, and two or three minutes for winding down. This might not sound like a lot and you may choose to gradually increase the amount of time you spend on each session, but all it takes is ten or fifteen minutes a day to start feeling a difference. If you can't set aside fifteen minutes each day with all your other responsibilities, just do what you can.

It is best to do your exercises on an empty stomach but don't be overzealous about this. There's no point in trying to do an effective yoga session if your tummy is rumbling. As a general rule it's sensible to wait at least an hour after eating before doing any yoga.

One of the nice things about yoga is that you can do it indoors or outside. Try to find somewhere relaxing and secluded enough for you not to be interrupted. If there is no carpet, place a folded blanket or rug on the floor. Never practise yoga on a mattress. Wear loose, comfortable clothing, take off jewellery and glasses, and remove your shoes. You might want to keep your socks on so your toes are warm.

Warm-Up/Cool-Down

As with any form of exercise, take a couple of minutes to stretch your muscles then lie flat on your back with your feet a couple of feet apart. The palms of your hands should face upwards, your arms at a 45-degree angle to your body. This is perhaps the most important of all the yoga positions, the **shavasana** or 'Corpse Position'. Breathe deeply from your abdomen. Feel your abdomen rise and fall gently with each breath. After a few deep breaths you are ready to start your yoga session.

At the end of each session take a few minutes to relax in the Corpse Position and adjust yourself to the outside world again, gradually waking yourself up to its sounds and sensations. If you are happy and settled in this position, stay here for as long as time permits. The Corpse Position at the beginning and end of each yoga session is a vital part of your routine and it shouldn't be missed.

Mountain Pose

The most basic building block of yoga from which many standing poses begin is the Mountain Pose, **tadasana**, literally 'straight as a mountain'. It is the most rock solid and firm of all the asanas. It is easier to achieve equilibrium and stability with this than with most other poses and you should learn to hold this pose before moving on to any of the more advanced ones. It also has the advantage of being one of the few asanas you can practise almost any time, anywhere.

1. Put your feet together, pointing your toes forward. Hang your arms by your sides, the palms facing inwards towards your body.
2. Imagine your body is suspended from a piano wire attached to the crown of your head. This will make your posture upright and erect and you should feel your spine and the back of your neck lengthening.
3. Now lift your toes off the ground and slowly place them back on the ground again. You will feel the arches of your feet lift as your toes lift. Maintain this feeling of the lift in your arches as you put your toes back down, and feel the lift all the way up your entire body.
4. Pull your thigh muscles upwards and lift the front of your body.
5. Relax your muscles. Relax your hands and face.
6. Hold this pose for as long as you feel comfortable. Feel

the strength, solidity and balance of it. Try to become one with the pose and feel the silence.

Breathing

It is important that you master at least one of the basic postures of yoga before you become overly conscious of your breathing. Your objective is to find peace within at least one pose. Once you have achieved this, when you have reached a point of equilibrium where staying still and sustaining the pose is easy and natural, you can begin focusing on your breath.

Breathing is life. In yoga it is known as **pranayama**. In the yogic tradition your breath is seen as the means by which life is extended from your spiritual being to your physical body (**prana** is 'life force,' **ayama** means 'to stretch or extend'). Breathing is the vital link between the physical and spiritual aspects of yoga.

The rules of breathing during yoga are simple. Don't take huge breaths and don't hold your breath – just breathe normally. Breathe through the nose unless you have a cold, hay fever or another sinus problem. Ten minutes in the Mountain Pose, breathing correctly, will give you a better idea of what yoga is all about.

You may like to try combining yoga with one of the meditation exercises we explored in the chapter on meditation. You can meditate while in the Corpse Position or while holding the Mountain Pose, but take it a step at a time. Master posture, breathing and meditation separately before putting them all together. Effective yoga is all about combining these three elements.

Yogic Posture

The celebrated yogi Patanjalin describes a successful yogic posture as being both steady and comfortable. Whether you join a class or learn yoga through a video, achieving 'steady and comfortable' takes practice. Every position contains an 'edge', the point beyond which you cannot comfortably go – for the time being anyway. Linger around this point with each posture, holding the position for as long as you can. This is the exact point where yoga draws its power. Strike a balance between pushing yourself out of the comfort-zone but not crossing over into pain. Yoga is all about balance, not extremes. This is worth remembering in your yoga class – yoga is not a competitive sport.

There are certain movements or postures which may work for others but not for you, so listen to your body. If you find a position too painful, don't do it, no matter how basic or 'easy' it is supposed to be.

If you are learning on your own from a tape or video, become fairly proficient at one posture before attempting to move on to the next. Spend entire sessions concentrating on each of the most basic postures, beginning with the standing positions before trying the balance poses or the floor posi-tions. If you don't learn to stand properly all the other positions will be unbalanced and out of alignment. This is the equivalent of learning scales when you first take up the piano. There is little point in trying to bash out a concerto when you haven't yet grasped the basics. Learn them, prac-tise them, master them, a few simple postures to begin with, then gradually expand your repertoire.

Your objective is to find equilibrium within each pose. The

yogic word for posture – asana – comes from the Sanskrit meaning 'to stay', and that's all it is. With any yoga pose you will reach a point of balance where staying still and sustaining the pose is easy and natural, where it feels 'right'. When you reach this point stay within the pose for as long as is comfortable. Try to become one with the pose and feel the silence. With correct breathing and mindfulness you will find peace within. It's that simple. As a general rule, the more challenging or difficult the pose the greater the inner peace once that asana has eventually been mastered.

Yoga is all about balance: reaching a point of equilibrium in an asana; getting the right balance between pushing the boundaries of comfort whilst avoiding pain; sustaining a balanced position for as long as feels natural; achieving physical and emotional equilibrium; and finding samadhi – equilibrium of the mind. Extensions are complemented by contractions, back bending postures are balanced by forward bending postures, inversions are followed by upright positions. A typical yoga workout is perfectly balanced.

Yoga Bytes

You can practise yoga 'bytes' at almost any time of the day. There are any number of breathing, stretching or facial exercises which you can do while you are waiting for the kettle to boil, sitting in traffic or waiting for a phone call. You might like to try a few moments of yoga instead of a cup of coffee mid-morning. Yoga is far more energizing!

The Yogic Diet

Central to the yogic tradition is the lifestyle which comes with the practice of yoga. Yogis see the body as a vehicle for the soul. It has certain needs if both are to function properly. Few, if any, Indian yogis are meat eaters. They believe in the idea of extending the circle of compassion to all living creatures and eating meat is seen to be in direct conflict with this belief. Food is fuel and a natural, simple, wholesome vegetarian diet is the best fuel there is.

Summary

To summarize: There are three aspects to yoga: body control, breath control and mind control. You may wish to dispense with mind control, as many Westerners do, but then it ceases to be yoga. The whole point of yoga is to use body postures and breathing to achieve mental equilibrium.

Begin with some basic postures, such as the Mountain Pose. Learn them, practise them, and master them.

Now master your breathing while holding a pose. Easy as this may seem, changing a lifelong habit of quick, short breaths may take a little time. After a few seconds of proper breathing, though, you will begin to feel the benefits.

When you have mastered your body and your breath you can move on to mastering your mind. Concentrate on visualization and breath counting as stepping stones towards 'no thought' meditation during your yoga practice.

Once you feel that you are successfully practising all three of these vital elements together, you can start to expand your repertoire of postures.

Sun Salutation

The Sun Salutation may be seen as a perfectly balanced sequence of poses – each position in the sequence stretches the body in a particular way and is counterbalanced by another position in the sequence which stretches the body in the opposite way. These positions alternately expand and contract your chest to encourage smooth and rhythmic breathing.

1. Stand upright with your legs straight, knees and feet together and palms touching in front of your chest. Distribute your weight evenly. Inhale deeply and exhale.
2. Inhaling, raise your arms above your head and lean backwards, arching your back from the waist.
3. Exhaling, drop your upper body downwards from the waist, so that your head and chest are pressing against your knees with your hands on the floor. (Bend your knees if necessary.)
4. Inhaling, extend one leg backwards as far as you can extend it, with your knee touching the ground. Arch your back, lift your chin, and look up.
5. Holding your breath, push your other leg back so that your legs are both fully extended behind you. Support your weight on your hands and toes. Keeping your head and spine in line, look down to the floor.
6. Exhaling, lower your knees, then your chest, and then your forehead, so that they are all touching the ground. Keep your hips up and your toes curled under.
7. Inhaling, lower your hips to the ground, arch your back

and point your toes, keeping your legs together. Relax your shoulders and tilt your head up and back.

8. Exhaling, lift your hips so that your body assumes an inverted V shape. Tuck your toes under, press your heels down and push your shoulders back.

9. Inhaling, extend one leg back in a mirror image of position 4.

10. Exhaling, bring your other leg forward and drop your body from the waist, mirroring position 3.

11. Inhaling, arch back from the waist, as in position 2.

12. Exhaling slowly, resume an upright position with your arms resting at your sides. Relax, with your weight distributed evenly between your two feet. Now repeat the sequence, beginning with the other leg.

The postures of the Sun Salutation, when smoothly linked together and repeated 12 times, limber the body in preparation for a yoga session. Try four 'rounds' of the exercise and gradually increase this over several weeks to 12.

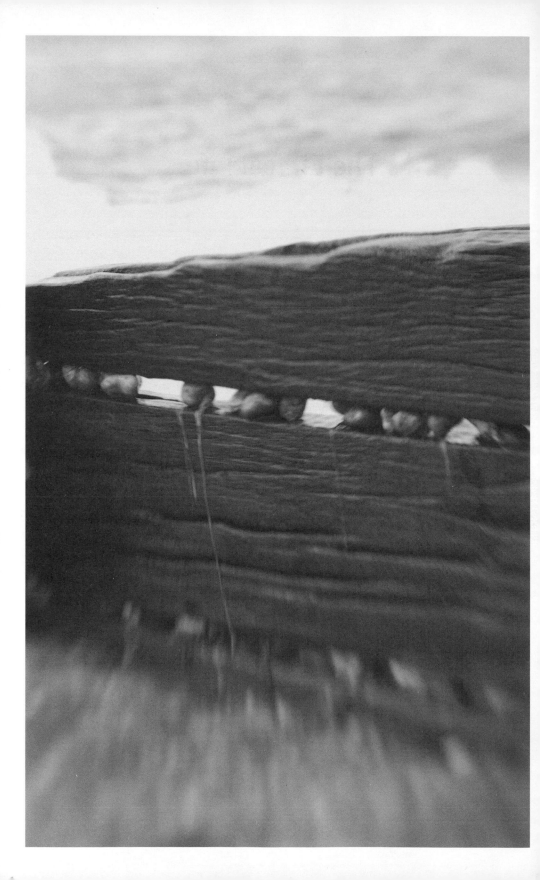

The Ethical Life

If, by the time you read this, you have undertaken just 30% of the suggestions outlined in *Life Balance* you won't need us to tell you that you have experienced a shift for the better in your attitude and outlook on life, and in your sense of fulfilment, too. Contrary to popular opinion, happiness is not an elusive concept . . . if you are prepared to work for it!

Of course, our whole society would be radically different if we had all been brought up learning how to look after our relationships, our finances, our bodies, minds and spirits. Instead of chasing after the next buck we would all recognize and value feeling good **within** and alter our priorities accordingly.

Such a fundamental shift in society's values is a long way off. All any individual can do is to change their own way of thinking and behaving so that they feel better about themselves. The interesting thing about this is that it is the best way to promote any lifestyle.

Heather: *Nothing validates an outlook on life more than to be full of life and vitality yourself.*

Personal Responsibility

None of us can hope to feel good about ourselves unless we live a life which respects our true values. As human beings we have certain rights which protect our welfare and security and upon which we all depend. With these rights comes an equal measure of personal responsibility. We have the right not to be harmed or injured by others and with this comes a responsibility not to do harm. We have the right to be treated with decency and fairness and in return we should be fair and decent in our dealings with others.

Do we treat our friends, family and colleagues fairly, with understanding, and do we pay regard to their needs? Does this treatment extend to strangers whose paths we cross, to animals, and to the planet which sustains us? There's not much point in being pleasant to your neighbours if you are endorsing corporations with abysmal human rights records by buying their goods. Buying fur for fashion when the animal in question has been abused all its life makes a mockery of cuddling the family dog. Personal responsibility isn't just about being nice to those who are close to us.

Ethical Eating

All of the food we eat comes at a cost, not just in terms of the money we pay for it but in terms of its impact on the world around us. It is clear that packing food full of unnatural chemicals and intensively rearing animals for food with little or no concern for their welfare is wrong.

Ben: *The only thing which will change this is pressure from the consumer – i.e., you. All retail outlets – from market stalls to international supermarket chains – are driven entirely by what the individual consumer wants, so vote with your wallet. Ten years ago, most supermarket chains wouldn't touch free-range or organic produce with a barge-pole; nowadays, these constitute a significant part of their output. Refuse to buy goods which are unethical and you will be making a difference. Anyone who thinks that an individual cannot make a difference has never shared a bed with a mosquito!*

It is a common fallacy that slaughter is carefully regulated in the UK. It is poorly governed and plagued by animal abuse. Meat inspectors – whose job it is to ensure proper handling and stunning of animals – focus primarily on meat hygiene. They therefore devote most of their attention to that part of the abattoir where animals are processed, rather than where they are slaughtered. Viva! has filmed in abattoirs across the UK and estimates that many millions of animals have their throats cut while fully conscious.

Heather: *Time and again undercover investigations by organizations such as People for the Ethical Treatment of Animals (PETA), Viva!, Animal Aid, and Compassion in World Farming have demonstrated that animal welfare regulations are routinely ignored. Every year in the United Kingdom more than 900 million mammals and birds are slaughtered for food. That is equivalent to more than 28 living creatures being slaughtered per second, every second, 365 days per year. Millions more die of stress, suffocation, disease or injuries in the process. The huge numbers of animals being raised and killed for food makes* *it impossible to treat them in a way the average person would consider humane.*

Recent research by Compassion in World Farming has shown that intensively reared farm animals such as cows, pigs, goats and chickens are capable of strong emotions such as pain, fear and even anxiety about the future. Christine Nicol, Professor of Animal Welfare at Bristol University, says that animals may be so emotionally similar to humans that welfare laws need to be reconsidered. 'Remarkable cognitive abilities and cultural innovations have been revealed,' she said. 'Our challenge is to teach others that every animal we intend to eat or use is a complex individual, and to adjust our farming culture accordingly.' (*Sunday Times*, 27 February, 2005, 'The Secret Life of Moody Cows' by Jonathan Leake, Science Editor). Research has documented that cows within a herd forge friendships with other cows that they like to spend most of their time with, often licking or grooming each other. They can also dislike other cows in the herd and they have been known to bear grudges for periods of months or even years. The notion that animals are incapable of thought and feeling has been conclusively disproved.

Eating meat leaves behind an environmental toll that generations to come will have to deal with. Since 1950, half of all the world's rain forests have been destroyed to make way for grazing animals. Tribal people are forced to move on as their habitat is sold off to the meat industry, and after just six or seven years of grazing, the soil is so damaged that it can no longer even support grass. In the UK, hedgerows are being destroyed for the same reason – intensive farming.

In addition to the ethical questions there is also sound

184

financial sense in being a vegetarian. A meat-based diet generally costs more than a vegetarian one. Furthermore, vegetarians are less likely to suffer from obesity, high blood pressure, arthritis, gallstones, constipation and many other ailments.

A vegetarian diet can be delicious and to prove it there are plenty of 'foodie' vegetarians out there. Many people are surprised at how easy the transition from meat eating to vegetarianism can be. You might want to treat yourself to a visit to a proper Italian delicatessen where you can buy the most exquisite handmade pastas, sauces, olives, roasted vegetables and breads – none of them costing the earth. The money you save by not buying meat should be spent on some really delicious, high-quality food.

Heather: *If you find you are craving a bacon butty, I challenge you to tell the difference between the taste of a slither of pig flesh and the soya alternative! When guests eat my BLT they always say, 'So you don't mind cooking meat for non-veggies then?'*

Most supermarkets have a range of vegetarian dishes and there are health food shops in abundance in most towns or cities where you will find row upon row of wonderful products that you never knew existed: veggie burgers, sausages, pasties, pies and imitation-meat products that can be used in your favourite recipes, as well as vegetarian foods that have been popular in other countries for many years such as falafel, tempeh or seitan.

More and more people are choosing a vegetarian way of life. 'Nothing will benefit human health and increase chances for survival of life on Earth as much as the evolution to a vegetarian diet,' wrote Albert Einstein. There are now more than four million vegetarians in the UK alone who agree with him.

Ethical Shopping

Where half the world's population does not have access to safe drinking water; where the work that people do is unfairly reflected in the wage they are paid for it; where our environment is threatened by the destruction of the ozone layer; where whole species of wildlife become extinct each year; we are responsible not only for what we do but for what we fail to speak out about. Each of us has a voice, both literally and in terms of how and where we buy our goods.

Companies of any size depend entirely upon the goodwill and support of their customers. The key to progress lies in the power of intelligent consumer action: ethical shoppers are beginning to make informed decisions about which consumer brands are best for the planet, for animals and for other people around the globe.

We can all make a difference, simply by modifying our spending patterns. By choosing one brand of coffee over another we can help to support the farmers who grow it rather than channelling our money into an organization which has little or no concern for human rights. Similarly, we can make an informed decision about what sort of washing-up liquid we use by avoiding one which damages the environment and opting instead for another which is dedicated to reducing pollution.

Ethical Consumer magazine puts the case clearly: 'Buying ethical products sends support directly to progressive companies working to improve the status quo, while at the same time depriving others that abuse for profit. For example, when you buy an eco-washing-up liquid you're giving its manufacturer the funds it needs to invest in clean technology and advertise its products for a wider market. At the same time, you're no longer buying your old liquid, so its manufacturer loses business and will perhaps change its ways.'

The problem, of course, is knowing where to begin and where to turn for ongoing information. It is great news that information on ethical shopping **is** constantly changing – it shows that we, the buying public, really are making a difference. There are a number of magazines, books and websites which are dedicated to helping consumers make informed decisions about their spending. Foremost amongst these are *The Good Shopping Guide* (www.thegoodshopping guide.co.uk), The Ethical Company Organisation (www.ethical-company-organisation.org), *Ethical Consumer* magazine (www.ethicalconsumer.org) and www.viva.org.uk. If you don't have access to the internet you can find copies of *The Good Shopping Guide* in all good bookshops and most major libraries.

We have one final exercise for you before you finally put down this book. Take the phone off the hook, kick off your shoes and make yourself comfortable. Take a few deep breaths. Picture yourself – the old, outdated you who controlled your life up until the time you started considering *Life Balance*. See your old self sitting as you are now, in the same chair and in the same position. Now picture the outer layers of the Old You – your clothes, skin and hair – peeling away like a snakeskin to reveal a fresh, new person underneath. Notice your clear conscience, fresh complexion, sparkling eyes, gentle smile and shiny hair. Take all of this in carefully, for this is the person you will be living with for the rest of your life, the real You.

References

Billeston, Jennie. (2001). *Secrets of Yoga*. London, Dorling Kindersley.

Budilovsky, Joan, and Adamson, Eve. (1999). *The Complete Idiot's Guide To Meditation*. New York, USA, Alpha Books.

Budilovsky, Joan, and Adamson, Eve. (2003). *The Complete Idiot's Guide To Yoga*. New York, USA, Alpha Books.

Campbell, T. Colin. (2005). *The China Study*. Dallas, BenBella Books.

Clayton, Emily. (2003). *Space Clearing*. CA, USA, Thunder Press.

Collins, Josephine. (2003). *Detox For Life: Purify Your Mind, Body and Soul.* London, Ryland Peters & Small.

Cousins, Barbara. (1997). *Cooking Without*. London, Thorsons.

Greener, Mark. (1996). *Which? Guide To Managing Stress*. London, Which? Books.

Hanh, Thich Nhat. (1991). *Peace Is Every Step*. London, Random House.

Hanh, Thich Nhat. (1991). *The Miracle Of Mindfulness*. London, Arrow Books.

Hewitt, James. (1978). *Teach Yourself Meditation*. London, Teach Yourself Books.

Jones, Annie. (1998). *Yoga In A Nutshell*. London, Element Books.

Kenton, Leslie. (1996). *Boost Energy*. London, Vermilion.

Kenton, Leslie. (1996). *Sleep Deep*. London, Vermilion.

Kirsta, Alix. (1986). *The Book Of Stress Survival*. London, HarperCollins.

Lindenfield, Gael. (1986). *Assert Yourself*. London, Thorsons.

Lindenfield, Gael. (1989). *Super Confidence*. London, Thorsons.

Lindenfield, Gael. (1995). *Self Esteem*. London, Thorsons.

Manktelow, James. (2004). *Make Time For Success!: The Time Management Masterclass*. London, Mind Tools Corporation.

Ozaniec, Naomi. (1997). *101 Essential Tips: Everyday Meditation.* London, Dorling Kindersley.

Robinson, Lynne, and Napper, Howard, with Brien, Caroline. (2002). *Intelligent Exercise With Pilates and Yoga*. London, Macmillan.

Robinson, Lynne, and Thomson, Gordon. (2005). *A New Body In 4 Weeks*. London, Pan Books.

Roland, Paul. (2002). *Meditation*. London, HarperCollins.

Scrivner, Jane. (1999*). Detox Your Life*. London, Judy Piatkus.

Scrivner, Jane. (1999*). Detox Your Mind*. London, Judy Piatkus.

Sivananda Yoga Vedanta Center. (1993). *Learn Yoga in a Weekend*. London, Dorling Kindersley.

Sivananda Yoga Vedanta Center. (1996). *Yoga Mind & Body*. London, Dorling Kindersley.

Smith, Patricia, Kalnitsky, Eugene, and MacFarlane, Muriel. (2002). *The Complete Idiot's Guide to Wellness*. New York, USA, Alpha Books.

Stacey, Sarah, and Fairley, Josephine. (2004). *The 21st Century Beauty Bible*. Leicester, Silverdale Books.

References

Walters, J. Donald. (1997). *Secrets of Meditation*. CA, USA, Crystal Charity Publishers.

Weil, Andrew. (2000). *Eating Well For Optimum Health*. London, Warner Books.

Williamson, Marianne. (2003). *Everyday Grace: Having Hope, Finding Forgiveness and Making Miracles.* London, Bantam.

Wilson, Paul. (1999). *The Big Book of Calm*. London, Michael Joseph.

The following websites have also been extremely useful in researching this book:

www.drbass.com

www.learningmeditation.com

www.meditationcenter.com

www.mindtools.com

www.moneysavingexpert – Martin Lewis's excellent website, definitely worth a visit

www.MoreToLife.org

www.tm.org

www.viva.org.uk

www.wccm.org

www.well-net.com

Acknowledgements

With special thanks to: Paul, Fiona, Sonya Mills, Jonny Geller, Doug Kean, Kate Adams, Louise Moore, Anya Noakes, Dr Neal Barnard, Dawn Carr at PETA, Lee Eastman, Sarah Campion, the amazing Dolley/Bond/Blackham Family, James Lucas, James Barber, Philip Watson, Mando Watson, Vivien Noakes, Michael Noakes, Alison Gillow, Lillian Shapiro, Lionel Shapiro, Andrew Parr, Philip Bergman, Charles Palmer, Darren Darnborough, Eileen Noakes, Francine Fletcher, Steve Fletcher, Graeme Grant, Ivan Hatvany, Joyce Treasure, Melanie Oliver, the wonderful team at Melrose & Morgan who have given us sustenance, Yvette Brown and The Typing Pool, Clare Latimer, Gladys Cacouratos, Randy North, Philip Sallon, Steve Gough, Valerie Daniel, Vida Box, Mike Mayhew, Margie Finchell, Azi Ahmed, Miranda Holden, Ande Adeniji, Richard Nickols, Shakuntala Polly Devi-Callaghan, Carola Byring, Jeanette Woolley, Vyvyan Chatterjie, everyone at Studio One, Louise Lucas, Ella Barber, Oliver and, of course, Harvey.